Therapeutic Stretching

Hands-On Guides for Therapists

Jane Johnson, MCSP, MSc

The London Massage Company

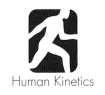

Human Kinetics

Library of Congress Cataloging-in-Publication Data

Johnson, Jane, 1965-
 Therapeutic stretching / Jane Johnson.
   p. ; cm. -- (Hands-on guides for therapists)
 ISBN 978-1-4504-1275-9 (print) -- ISBN 1-4504-1275-0 (print)
 I. Title. II. Series: Hands-on guides for therapists.
 [DNLM: 1. Muscle Stretching Exercises. 2. Musculoskeletal Diseases--rehabilitation. 3.
Physical Therapy Modalities. WB 541]

 613.7'182--dc23

                                          2011045623
 ISBN-10: 1-4504-1275-0 (print)
 ISBN-13: 978-1-4504-1275-9 (print)

Copyright © 2012 by Jane Johnson

Acquisitions Editors: Loarn D. Robertson, PhD, and Karalynn Thomson; **Developmental Editor:** Amanda S. Ewing; **Assistant Editors:** Kali Cox and Derek Campbell; **Copyeditor:** Patricia L. MacDonald; **Graphic Designer:** Nancy Rasmus; **Graphic Artist:** Dawn Sills; **Cover Designer:** Keith Blomberg; **Photographer (cover):** Neil Bernstein; **Photographer (interior):** Neil Bernstein; **Photo Asset Manager:** Laura Fitch; **Visual Production Assistant:** Joyce Brumfield; **Photo Production Manager:** Jason Allen; **Art Manager:** Kelly Hendren; **Associate Art Manager:** Alan L. Wilborn; **Illustrations:** © Human Kinetics; **Printer:** Versa Press

Printed in the United States of America   10 9 8 7 6 5 4 3 2 1

The paper in this book is certified under a sustainable forestry program.

Human Kinetics
Website: www.HumanKinetics.com

United States: Human Kinetics
P.O. Box 5076
Champaign, IL 61825-5076
800-747-4457
e-mail: humank@hkusa.com

Canada: Human Kinetics
475 Devonshire Road Unit 100
Windsor, ON N8Y 2L5
800-465-7301 (in Canada only)
e-mail: info@hkcanada.com

Europe: Human Kinetics
107 Bradford Road
Stanningley
Leeds LS28 6AT, United Kingdom
+44 (0) 113 255 5665
e-mail: hk@hkeurope.com

Australia: Human Kinetics
57A Price Avenue
Lower Mitcham, South Australia 5062
08 8372 0999
e-mail: info@hkaustralia.com

New Zealand: Human Kinetics
P.O. Box 80
Torrens Park, South Australia 5062
0800 222 062
e-mail: info@hknewzealand.com

e5499

The first workshop I ever ran was called Effective Stretching. This book is dedicated to the handful of therapists who took part in that workshop and to the hundreds who have since attended my stretching workshops in order to gain extra therapeutic skills. Your questions and comments have helped inform my understanding of how and for whom stretching is a useful treatment intervention.

Contents

PART III   Implementing Your Stretches

PART IV   Stretching Routines

Series Preface

Massage may be one of the oldest therapies still used today. At present more therapists than ever before are practicing an ever-expanding range of massage techniques. Many of these techniques are taught through massage schools and within degree courses. Our need now is to provide the best clinical and educational resources that will enable massage therapists to learn the required techniques for delivering massage therapy to clients. Human Kinetics has developed the Hands-On Guides for Therapists series with this in mind.

The Hands-On Guides for Therapists series provides specific tools of assessment and treatment that fall well within the realm of massage therapists but may also be useful for other bodyworkers, such as osteopaths and fitness instructors. Each book in the series is a step-by-step guide to delivering the techniques to clients. Each book features a full-colour interior packed with photos illustrating every technique. Tips provide handy advice to help you adjust your technique, and the Client Talk boxes contain examples of how the techniques can be used with clients who have particular problems. Throughout each book are questions that enable you to test your knowledge and skill, which will be particularly helpful if you are attempting to pass a qualification exam. We've even provided the answers too!

You might be using a book from the Hands-On Guides for Therapists series to obtain the required skills to help you pass a course or to brush up on skills you learned in the past. You might be a course tutor looking for ways to make massage therapy come alive with your students. This series provides easy-to-follow steps that will make the transition from theory to practice seem effortless. The Hands-On Guides for Therapists series is an essential resource for all those who are serious about massage therapy.

Preface

As therapists and fitness professionals, many of us have worked with clients recovering from musculoskeletal injuries such as sprained ankles, pulled calves or tennis elbows. We have certainly helped clients suffering muscular tension in the form of tight hamstrings, a stiff neck or lumbar pain. For all these kinds of conditions, stretching is often recommended as part of the treatment solution in addition to modalities such as massage. This book provides a comprehensive range of stretches to help you safely and effectively treat clients rehabilitating from common musculoskeletal conditions.

Being able to safely stretch a client as part of your massage, physical therapy or fitness training programme is a valuable skill. So too is the ability to provide advice on the sorts of stretches clients might do at home as part of their rehabilitation from injury or to help them manage muscular pain or joint stiffness. In addition, modification of standard stretches is essential when treating people after injury or when working with special populations such as elderly clients. This guide will help you apply passive stretches in a confident and competent manner, teaching you how to best position your clients and which sorts of handholds to use when applying stretches to clients with musculoskeletal problems. Photographs throughout provide visual prompts to help get you started if you have never performed passive stretches before.

The book is organized into four parts. In part I you learn how to get started and prepare for stretching. Here you are encouraged to consider both why we need therapeutic stretching and the challenge of designing a stretching protocol. The rationale for stretching after musculoskeletal injury is outlined along with general safety guidelines, plus a full list is given of the musculoskeletal conditions covered and for which this book provides stretches. This part of the book also sets out the 10 steps to follow as you prepare a stretching programme.

In part II you will learn to differentiate between passive, active and advanced forms of stretching such as muscle energy technique (MET) and soft tissue release (STR). The advantages and disadvantages of each are explored in terms of how easy they are to apply, on which parts of the body they may be used and for which types of musculoskeletal injuries they are most appropriate.

Part III is the main part of the book and is divided into three chapters. Each of these chapters focuses on a different section of the body and the kinds of musculoskeletal conditions that are appropriate for rehabilitative stretching. Chapter 5 on the lower limb covers the foot and ankle, knee and leg, and hip and thigh and includes stretches for conditions such as a sprained ankle, shin splints and runner's knee as well as treatments for clients who report having tight calves or hamstrings. Chapter 6 provides stretches for the upper limb—the shoulder, elbow, wrist, hand and fingers. Here you will find information for helping clients with conditions such as adhesive capsulitis, lateral epicondylitis and stiff wrists. Chapter 7 focuses on stretches relating to the back and neck and includes advice on the kinds of stretches suitable for treating clients who are kyphotic, suffer low back pain or a stiff neck or are recovering from whiplash injury.

Each of the chapters in part III includes both active and passive stretches; the main focus is on passive stretching (i.e., the stretches that may be performed safely by a sports massage therapist, sports rehabilitator, physical therapist or osteopath with a client sitting or lying on a treatment couch). Active stretches are included so that you may select from these in order to create a stretching programme for your clients to use at home.

Part IV sets out the stretches from the main part of the book in the form of routines. Here, illustrations from earlier chapters have been collated so you can perform a series of stretches in the prone, supine or seated position. This part will help you practise and become confident in applying the stretches without having to turn a subject from one position to another. As with other titles in the Hands-On Guide for Therapists series, the quick questions appearing at the end of most chapters will ensure you have grasped the main ideas being presented.

I began writing this book knowing you cannot please all of the people all of the time, and that to provide information on all stretches in all positions for every type of client, as well as cover a variety of musculoskeletal conditions, was not going to be possible in a book of this size. However, I hope the stretches that are included will be useful to many readers. These are stretches I have found particularly helpful in my own work as both a physiotherapist and sport massage therapist. Many of the stretches I used when working as a personal trainer. Please share this information with your colleagues, and as with the other books in this series (*Soft Tissue Release*, *Deep Tissue Massage* and *Postural Assessment*), please feel free to contact me with your comments and suggestions.

Acknowledgements

I would like to thank Karalynn Thomson, acquisitions editor at Human Kinetics, for considering and approving this book, originally submitted as *Stretch Your Clients*. Thanks also to Amanda Ewing, who has done a splendid job in editing the manuscript, her third title with me to date. Thanks must also go to copyeditor Patricia MacDonald, graphic designer Nancy Rasmus and graphic artist Dawn Sills. Thank you also to photographer Neil Bernstein; Doug Nelson (therapist model); and Bob McLeese, Norma Hollen, Chelsea Reynolds and Zach McClughen, who posed for the photographs.

Getting Started With Therapeutic Stretching

If you have been wanting to know how to incorporate stretching into your treatments, or if you are curious as to how to provide safe stretches for clients to use at home, here in part I you will find two chapters containing everything you need to help get you started. Chapter 1 lists some of the reasons people are already using stretching and explains what makes *therapeutic* stretching special. This chapter lists the pathologies (such as frozen shoulder, sprained ankle, stiff low back) for which you will find stretches in later chapters of the book, along with the reasons these stretches have been suggested. As you would expect, there are also some guidelines to help you apply stretches safely when treating clients with musculoskeletal conditions.

Chapter 2 provides 10 easy steps to help you decide how to plan, implement and review a stretching programme. There are examples of the kinds of goals you might wish to set with your clients, the advantages and disadvantages of providing stretches in various environments, plus ideas for measuring the effectiveness of a stretching programme. This chapter also contains information on the use of therapeutic stretching when working with special populations. The three groups that have been selected are elderly clients, pregnant women and athletes.

At the end of each chapter are five quick questions, useful if you want to check what you remember as you progress through the book.

Introduction to Therapeutic Stretching

This chapter describes therapeutic stretching, the rationale for its use and why you might want to consider using it with clients. Included is an overview of the musculoskeletal injuries and conditions for which you will find stretches in later chapters of this book, along with a brief description of each condition. The section on why people stretch leads to a discussion concerning the challenge of designing a stretching protocol for the rehabilitation and treatment of clients with common musculoskeletal conditions. This chapter also sets out the general stretching recommendations for each of the musculoskeletal conditions covered in this book (e.g., sprains, strains, stiff joints) along with the rationale for these recommendations. The general safety guidelines at the end of this chapter will help you feel confident incorporating stretching into your practice.

What Is Therapeutic Stretching?

Throughout this book, the term *therapeutic stretching* refers to any stretching that is performed with the intention of deliberately facilitating an improvement in a person's physical or psychological well-being. It could be argued that all forms of stretching are therapeutic. The difference here is in the intention of the person performing or assisting the stretches. Here we advocate the use of stretching not simply as a pre- or post-exercise habit but as a means of bringing about a specific therapeutic outcome. With therapeutic stretching, appropriate stretches are identified, modified where necessary, well planned and well executed, and their effects are monitored.

The Need for Therapeutic Stretching

One disadvantage of some stretching books is they assume the people for whom the stretches are recommended are fit and healthy and flexible enough to get into what are sometimes quite challenging positions. Consider the popular image of someone dressed in fitness clothing performing a hamstring stretch: The person is standing on one leg, reaching over to touch the toes of the opposite foot, which is resting on a gatepost or park bench. This position necessitates not only a straight leg raise of at least 90 degrees but also the ability to place almost the full weight of the body onto the supporting leg whilst remaining balanced. Although we should avoid pigeonholing elderly people as being frail and physically incapacitated, it is fair to say that the minority of seniors would be able to get into such a position to stretch the hamstrings. Most older adults lose strength in their lower limb muscles and experience joint stiffness, and they often have poor balance. So, too, might a person recovering from a knee, ankle or foot injury. A standing hamstring stretch is therefore not the best stretch to recommend to this group of clients, and alternatives are needed.

How might we as therapists help seniors and clients rehabilitating musculoskeletal conditions reap the benefits of stretching? The answer lies in our ability to modify stretches. Physical therapists, sports therapists and fitness professionals are used to designing exercise programmes tailored to the individual. Similarly, we need to identify and to modify stretches so they may be applied in such a way as to be both effective and safe for older adults and those recovering from musculoskeletal conditions. We need to embrace the concept of therapeutic stretching.

Why Should I Incorporate Stretching Into My Practice?

One doesn't randomly employ the use of ice (cryotherapy), immobilization, cognitive behavioural therapy (CBT), manual lymphatic drainage or balance training in a treatment. These, as with all interventions, are selected by therapists on the basis of believing they will help bring about a specific treatment outcome. Stretching is a treatment intervention just as is rest, exercise, massage and ultrasound. Whether you incorporate stretches into a treatment depends on your objectives. For more on the kinds of objectives for which stretching might be appropriate, see pages 9 and 20.

Overview of Musculoskeletal Conditions Covered in This Book

Therapeutic Stretching is part of a series of books primarily—but not solely—for massage therapists. It is likely that a large proportion of readers will be providing massage to people within the general population, some working in private practices (rather than in hospitals), some preferring to treat specific client groups such as athletes or the elderly. A great many people are affected by conditions that produce adverse changes in their muscles, tendons, ligaments and the associated soft tissues (skin, connective tissue, sometimes neural and vascular structures), and sooner or later most massage therapists find themselves treating a client recovering from one of these conditions—a sprained ankle, torn hamstring or stiff neck, for example. The pathologies covered in this book (and the pages on which you can find suitable stretches in later chapters) have been grouped according to the category of condition into which they fall (e.g., strains, sprains, stiff joints). Use the page numbers listed in the sidebar Musculoskeletal Conditions to locate the conditions for which you require stretching ideas, or turn directly to the appropriate chapter for those conditions affecting the lower limb (chapter 5), the upper limb (chapter 6) and the trunk (chapter 7).

It is useful to quickly review each condition in order to understand the rationale behind the stretching recommendations set out in table 1.1 on page 12.

Musculoskeletal Conditions

Sprains
  Ankle sprain, page 54
  Wrist sprain, page 106

Strains
  Calf strain, page 63
  Hamstring strain, page 69
  Groin strain, page 75
  Rotator cuff strain, page 97
  Low back strain, page 125

Cramps
  In calf muscles, page 66
  In hamstring muscles, page 73
  In the neck (wry neck), page 115

Stiff muscles
  Tight calf, page 65
  Tight hamstrings, page 70
  Tight adductors, page 76
  Tight quadriceps, page 78
  Tight hip flexors, page 80
  Tight shoulder muscles (see adhesive capsulitis), page 89
  Tight neck muscles, page 120
  Tight chest muscles (see kyphotic postures), page 121

Stiff joints
  Ankle, page 59
  Shoulder, page 92
  Elbow, page 104
  Wrist/Fingers, page 107
  Neck, page 116

  Thorax (see kyphotic postures), page 121
  Lumbar spine, page 131

Tendon problems
  Achilles tendinopathies, page 56
  Supraspinatus tendinosis, page 99
  Lateral epicondylitis, page 102
  Medial epicondylitis, page 103

Fascia structures
  Plantar fasciitis, page 62
  Iliotibial band friction syndrome (runner's knee), page 82

Nerve compression
  Piriformis syndrome, page 83
  Carpal tunnel syndrome, page 109

After surgery
  Knee surgery, page 68
  Mastectomy, page 101

Other pathologies
  Ankle fracture, page 58
  Shin splints, page 64
  Osteoarthritis of the knee, page 66
  DOMS (delayed onset muscle soreness), page 85
  Adhesive capsulitis (frozen shoulder), page 89
  Shortened internal rotators of the humerus, page 95
  Whiplash, page 113
  Kyphotic postures, page 121
  Herniated disc, page 134

Sprains

A sprain is an acute injury involving the tearing of a ligament that would normally hold two or more bones together. Sprains are accompanied by damage to blood vessels, nerves and connective tissue and are graded according to the degree of fibre damage. Very generally, a grade I sprain indicates mild damage with just a few ligamentous fibres being torn, whereas a grade III sprain describes severe damage, with complete rupture of the ligament. A grade II sprain may be mild (less than 50 percent of fibres torn) or severe (more than 50 percent of fibres torn). The more severe the damage, the more severe the bleeding, swelling and pain. After severe sprains, a joint is less stable (with an increase in range of motion), yet range of motion is reduced in the acute stages because of swelling. A severe sprain may involve injury to bone, such as an avulsion fracture where the ligament is wrenched forcibly off the bone at the ligament's attachment point. Healing usually takes three to six weeks, and in severe cases the injured part may be immobilized for up to three weeks, resulting in a decreased range of motion and stiffening of the associated joint due to scar tissue formation and decreased synovial fluid. When pain subsides, the injury is described as sub-acute.

Strains

A strain is an acute injury involving the tearing of muscle fibres, the muscle's tendon, or both. As with sprains, this too may involve damage to blood vessels, nerves and connective tissues. There is usually more bleeding than with a sprain because muscles are more highly vascularized than ligaments. As with sprains, there are various grades of strain: mild, moderate or severe, each corresponding to the degree of fibre damage. Where there is complete rupture, function is impaired because the muscle can no longer generate force to pull a bone and move a body part. The more severe the damage, the more severe the bleeding, swelling and pain. Healing may take three to five weeks but can be much longer in the case of severe strains. As with sprains, when pain subsides the injury is described as sub-acute.

An important point to note with regard to both strains and sprains is that pain usually subsides long before healing is complete. This makes the potential for reinjury high if the client uses pain as a guide for deciding whether or not to use that body part. During therapeutic stretching, it is usually recommended that clients perform exercises or stretches that are *within their pain-free range*, using pain as a warning sign to stop the activity. This lessens the likelihood of reinjury.

Cramps

A cramp is a sudden, involuntary contraction in a muscle that is temporary but that can be very painful. The cause is unknown, although cramps are associated with peripheral vascular disease and may be precipitated by water and electrolyte disturbances. They are also reported by clients with hypotension or those taking certain medications. Muscles commonly reported to cramp are those of the feet, calf and hamstrings. This may occur during the night or after or during physical exertion. Sometimes muscles cramp when they have been held in a shortened position (an important point to note when stretching the antagonist muscle). Although they have less severe consequences than some of the other musculoskeletal conditions listed here, cramps are nevertheless annoying for those who suffer them, especially when they occur at night and disturb sleep or when they impair sporting performance.

Stiff Muscles

This term suggests an increase in muscle tone and commonly refers to muscles that a client reports as feeling tight or that on palpation feel more stiff to a therapist. Tension (i.e., an increase in tone) in muscles is therefore measureable both objectively (by the client) and subjectively (by the therapist). Tight muscles may be shorter than the norm when measured using a standard muscle length test. However, in some cases a client may report feelings of tightness in muscles (such as the hamstrings) that are found to be of a regular or even a greater length than normal when measured by a therapist. Therefore muscle length tests are useful but limited when used to assess what clients describe as 'tight' muscles. In *Therapeutic Stretching*, the term is used to mean the subjective sensation of tension described by most clients when they say they have 'tight calf muscles', for example, whether or not this is measureable as a decrease in range of motion in the joint or joints associated with a particular muscle or as a perceived increase in stiffness on palpation by a therapist.

Stiff Joints

Stiff joints are those that a client reports as feeling stiff or that on testing have a less than normal range of motion (ROM). Joints may be stiff for a variety of reasons. Stiffness may result from direct immobilization of a joint (e.g., in a brace or cast), from injury (such as a severe ankle sprain) or from immobilization of some other part of the associated limb (e.g., when the whole arm is kept in a sling after an elbow injury, and the shoulder joint stiffens too). Sometimes clients complain of stiffness resulting from a previous injury where there was little or no intervention and where function has been restored but limitations in range of motion remain. For example, without intervention, joints commonly stiffen temporarily after surgery to them. This may be a result of effusion within the joint and surrounding tissues or the formation of excessive amounts of scar tissue. In the case of adhesive capsulitis, the shoulder joint stiffens with no known cause.

Stretching is not appropriate for all the causes of stiff joints. For example, in ankylosing spondylitis, joints fuse together over time, and stretching them would not necessarily be an appropriate intervention because the joints are mechanically fused, and their range cannot be improved (other than with surgery). Clients suffering rheumatoid arthritis experience pain, swelling and stiffness in joints, especially the small joints of the fingers and toes. Stretching is contraindicated (as is massage) during inflammatory periods when the stretching could exacerbate the inflammation.

Tendon Problems

Painful conditions resulting from overuse of tendons fall within a group of pathologies known as tendinopathies. Most massage therapists know that -*itis* means 'inflammation'.

Inflammation of a tendon (identified by histopathological sampling of the tissue) is known as tendin*itis* (or tendon*itis*). Conditions such as lateral and medial epicondyl*itis* were initially thought to fall into this category but are now better described as being tendinosies. Tendinosies are tendon problems resulting from overuse and are very painful. Yet on microscopic examination, the tendon is found to have fewer inflammatory markers than expected, indicating that the healing process has been interrupted. Medial and lateral epicondylitis are therefore not true tendinitises because they lack certain cellular characteristics that are indicative of inflammation.

As with sprains and strains, pain associated with tendon problems usually subsides long before tendon damage is fully resolved and tissues fully repaired. People recovering from conditions affecting their tendons are therefore at risk of reinjury if they return to physical activity too soon.

Fascia Structures

Two common conditions believed to be the result of fascial changes are plantar fasciitis and iliotibial band friction syndrome (runner's knee). There is growing interest in treatments aimed specifically at bringing about changes in fascia, generally known as myofascial release techniques. One could argue that myofascial release falls into the category of therapeutic stretching as it involves the gentle, sustained traction of soft tissues and thus embodies an element of stretching that is used to bring about a specific therapeutic outcome.

Nerve Compression

Whilst this book does not cover the kinds of stretches specifically designed to relieve tension in neural structures (sometimes adapted from neural tension tests), it does include two conditions that involve compression of nerves: piriformis syndrome and carpal tunnel syndrome. Descriptions of these can be found in chapters 5 and 6, respectively.

After Surgery

There are many common surgical procedures. The stretches included here (for use with patients after mastectomy and knee surgery) have been selected in order to demonstrate how stretches might be used post-surgically for one upper limb condition and one lower limb condition. Stress and motion are believed to stimulate collagen to form a more functional alignment of collagen fibres and a more functional scar (whether or not this scar can be seen) after surgery. Yet it is important not to stretch too early in the repair process because collagen must be matured. Stretch too soon and you risk tearing the connective tissue apart as it is undergoing remodelling. This could tear the vascular bed and lead to an increase in bleeding and pain. Pain may lead to muscle spasm. This in turn leads to increased inflammation and a prolonged period of rehabilitation.

Other Pathologies

In addition to these easily classified conditions, *Therapeutic Stretching* includes others that do not fit easily into the previous categories but that are nevertheless very common.

These are shin splints, osteoarthritis of the knee and DOMS (delayed onset muscle soreness) (chapter 5); adhesive capsulitis (chapter 6); and whiplash and kyphotic postures (chapter 7). Information about each can be found in their respective chapters.

Why Do People Stretch?

Before we turn to the rationale for stretching to treat the conditions described in the previous section, it might be useful to ask why people stretch. The answers might provide the basis for your treatment objectives. Some of the reasons cited for the use of stretching include the following:

- To help maintain normal muscle functioning
- To help alleviate pain due to muscle tension
- To overcome cramping in muscles
- To maintain or improve range of motion in a joint
- To facilitate muscle healing
- To help correct postural imbalances
- To help minimize the development of scar tissue
- To influence psychological factors, such as to aid relaxation, maintain or improve motivation or stimulate a sense of well-being

Let's consider some of these in turn. Most mammals stretch after a period of immobility. Cats and dogs, for example, stretch after sleep, as do humans. If you have ever had to remain in a stationary position, unable to stretch, you will know that pain in your muscles soon develops as tension increases, impairing normal muscle functioning. Perhaps you have experienced this after a long drive, train ride or plane journey, or if you have ever been bedbound as a result of injury or illness. Many people report having to get out of bed at night to walk off a cramp in a calf muscle. It feels instinctive to stretch one's muscles when they start to hurt or cramp. Stretching is therefore often used simply as a means of relieving muscle tension, and some professionals believe it may be helpful in preventing the development of trigger points. Perhaps the unplanned daily stretching most of us do helps maintain normal muscle functioning?

Stretching is also commonly used therapeutically in a variety of settings. For example, it is used in hospitals by physical therapists to maintain or improve range of motion in a joint, something that is particularly important after immobilization. Or it might be used in an attempt to combat the effects of muscle spasm and contractures. It may be used as part of a post-surgery rehabilitation protocol to help with the realignment of collagen fibres, decreasing the development of disadvantageous scar tissue adhesions. It is also used by athletes, traditionally as part of a team warm-up or cool-down, and is inherent to exercise classes where it is used in a similar manner. Sports and remedial therapists employ stretching to help correct postural imbalance: Exercises are used to shorten and strengthen weak muscles; stretches are used to lengthen shortened ones.

There are also psychological factors to consider. Many people experience a sense of well-being when they have stretched, and this may explain the popularity of yoga classes. Believing that stretching lessens their likelihood of injury, many people also stretch before exercise as part of their psychological preparation. Stretching is some-times advocated as part of a relaxation routine or to decrease levels of anxiety. Active stretching places responsibility for body maintenance with the patients, thus empower-ing them with some degree of control in their own rehabilitation and as such may be justification for its inclusion in a treatment regime. Sometimes, physically active people sustain injuries that prevent them from training, interrupting the stretching routine they are used to performing. For such clients, lack of routine physical activity can lead to negative feelings. Therefore gentle stretches performed actively in the initial stages of rehabilitation may keep such clients motivated and engaged with their recovery.

As you can see, stretching is already widely used. If we are to employ stretching in a therapeutic setting, we simply need to be more clear about our objectives and goals. Read again the list of answers to the question of why people stretch. Could any of these be used as an appropriate treatment objective for your clients? Turn to page 21 in chapter 2 for more information about treatment objectives and matching goals.

The Challenge of Designing a Stretching Protocol

In chapters 5, 6 and 7 you will find stretches that are safe to use when treating clients recovering from common musculoskeletal conditions. One of the challenges in putting together this material is that there are no agreed protocols for the use of therapeutic stretching. Whilst conditions such as sprains and strains follow recognizable and mea-surable stages of repair, we do not know how to incorporate stretching to bring about the *best* recovery outcomes for each person. Lack of discrete protocols is due in part to the problems inherent to researching the many variables associated with the application of manual therapies. It is also made difficult because people vary in how they recover physically and emotionally from injury and illness, as well as differing in how fit and healthy they were before sustaining an injury. So whilst we can say when the application of stretching is *likely* to be advantageous or disadvantageous, many questions remain unanswered regarding the specific protocols that should be used.

For example, for each of the conditions listed in this book, we do not know for certain for how long a particular stretch should be applied, which stretches are best (active or passive stretches) or whether it matters when stretches are used (what time of day or night). Nor do we know whether there is a minimum length of time for which a stretching posture should be maintained (although holding a static stretch for 30 seconds may be the minimum time needed to bring about a lengthening of soft tissues) or how frequently stretching should be performed (once a week? once a day? once an hour?). Also, we do not know to what extent a person's psychological well-being affects the outcome of her participation in a stretching programme, only that it seems reasonable to assume that a person is more likely to adhere to a stretching programme if she is motivated to recover quickly and believes stretching will help rather than demotivated and lacking faith in stretching as a useful rehabilitation tool.

It is not clear when stretching should be performed in order to get the best results. If stretching is being used as part of a relaxation programme, it might be best carried out at the end of the day, before a person retires to bed. If it is being used as part of a rehabilitation programme, to increase range of motion in a joint, for example, it may be desirable to perform stretches at several intervals throughout the day rather than just once. Whilst it is unclear how frequently stretching should be performed, or for how long stretches should be held, little and often seems favourable for enhancing the chances of compliance, especially when providing stretches for clients after musculoskeletal injury. Prolonged, continuous stretching may be more beneficial than short, intermittent bursts of stretching when attempting to improve range of motion or treating stiff joints or tight muscles. However, this requires longer chunks of time and may decrease the likelihood of compliance.

It is because we lack distinct protocols for therapeutic stretching that it is so important to document our treatments and record positive (or negative) outcomes. Only in this way can we begin to amass enough information to help us make more informed decisions about the use of stretching in the future. For now, we need to rely on our understanding of general physiological repair processes after injury and make well-reasoned judgements on how stretching is applied.

The Rationale for Stretching After Musculoskeletal Injury

Let's now look at each of the musculoskeletal conditions covered in chapters 5, 6 and 7 and the stretching recommendations for each. This information is set out in table 1.1. You will find the rationale for each recommendation in the right-hand column of the table. Use this information to guide you when selecting appropriate stretches to use with clients after injury. As you know, all clients differ, and a stretch that is suitable for one may be unsuitable for another. Always consider how to modify your stretches to suit individual clients, and if in doubt, select the stretch that puts the least amount of tension on tissues.

For readers who wish to gain a greater understanding about the physiology of stretching and limitations to flexibility, *The Science of Flexibility* by Michael J. Alter (Human Kinetics 2004) is highly recommended.

General Safety Guidelines

In addition to the recommendations set out in the previous section, it is prudent to adhere to these general safety guidelines when planning to implement a stretching programme.

- Follow the protocol (if there is one) of the clinic, hospital or practice in which you work.
- Adhere to the guidelines set out by the body that governs your profession.
- Where there are no guidelines or protocol, use your professional judgement and clinical experience. Ask yourself, *Is what I am doing safe? Knowing what I know about this client and this particular musculoskeletal condition, is stretching likely to be advantageous or disadvantageous? Does it seem reasonable that the stretching intervention I am intending to use could contribute to the positive outcome I desire?* If your answers are positive, continue; if not, select an alternative treatment to stretching.

Table 1.1 Stretching Recommendations and Rationale

Common musculoskeletal condition	General stretching recommendations	Rationale
Sprains and strains: acute	All forms of stretching are contraindicated during the early stages of healing (even with very mild sprains).	Tissues are in a fragile state. Any form of stretching could potentially redamage tissues and delay the healing process.
Sprains and strains: sub-acute	With caution, begin a gentle active stretching programme sooner rather than later.	This may help with the realignment of collagen fibres in a manner that means disadvantageous fibrous adhesions are less likely to occur.
	Passive stretching is contraindicated.	The pain experienced by clients in the sub-acute state can be variable and not easily judged by the therapist. Employing a passive stretch may elongate tissues to a point that could accidently redamage them, something less likely to occur when clients do the stretch themselves; clients are better able to judge when they are approaching their pain threshold, at which point they should stop the stretch.
	Where possible, elevate the injured joint or limb.	Elevation assists venous and lymphatic drainage and thus reduces any swelling that would otherwise impair stretching.
	The client should avoid weight bearing through the affected joint or limb.	This lessens the likelihood of reinjury in the early stages of rehabilitation, when proprioception and balance may be impaired and injured tissues not strong enough to stabilize the joint.
	Use gentle active movements of the injured joint.	This facilitates stretching of surrounding tissues, plus a decrease in swelling, especially in injuries to the foot and ankle where the calf muscle assists in venous and lymphatic drainage.
	Maintain range of motion but only within the client's pain-free range.	Pain is likely to indicate that the client is causing reinjury. Performing stretches within the pain-free range lessens the likelihood of reinjury.
	Joint movements that are most easy to perform should be introduced first.	This will increase the likelihood of compliance (no one likes to perform any exercise he finds difficult) and is likely to result in greater progress than if stretches are difficult.

Common musculoskeletal condition	General stretching recommendations	Rationale
Muscle cramp	Active stretches are most useful at helping to overcome a cramp.	Contraction of the opposing muscle group produces inhibition in the muscles that are cramping and thus alleviates the cramp more quickly than passive stretching (which does not inhibit contraction of the cramping muscle). Also, a cramp is involuntary and often occurs at night or after physical exertion, when a therapist is not available to perform passive stretching.
	Passive stretches are sometimes helpful.	Cramping may occur in a patient during treatment such as massage and is commonly experienced after physical exertion. Passively stretching a cramping muscle produces an increase in pain in the short term (i.e., during the stretch) that gradually eases and is useful before or after sporting events or when clients are not able to stretch the muscle themselves.
Tight muscles: mild	Both active and passive stretches are useful.	Used daily, active or passive stretching may serve as a prophylactic to worsening joint stiffness in some clients.
Tight muscles: chronic	Both active and passive stretching may be useful for different reasons.	With active stretching, the client can use her body weight to facilitate the stretch, especially useful when muscles are chronically tight. Conversely, the effort of concentrating on the maintenance of the stretch position may increase muscle tone in some people, making it difficult to overcome chronic tightness. Passive stretching may enable a client to relax more fully than when she is performing stretches actively and may therefore result in an improved stretch. Arguably, chronically tight muscles must be stretched daily, and so active stretches may be more viable as they do not require a stretching partner.

»continued

»continued

Common musculoskeletal condition	General stretching recommendations	Rationale
Stiff joints: mild	Both active and passive stretches are useful to combat mild stiffness in joints.	The stretch chosen depends on whether or not a therapist is available and whether or not a client is able to perform active stretches himself. Sometimes stiff joints become less stiff when a patient resumes his normal daily activities or takes up an occupation that involves increasing the range of motion in the affected joint. The client may incorporate the use of his body weight to help stretch soft tissues around the stiff joint. Performing active stretches places responsibility for stretching with the client, something that may be desirable in a rehabilitative setting.
Stiff joints: chronic	Passive stretches may be better for treating joints of the lower limbs.	Where a client has not been bearing weight on a limb for a period of time and may have lost her sense of balance, stretches in standing are likely to be unsafe. Passive stretches are helpful when a client cannot comfortably get into the position necessary to perform a stretch.
Tendinopathies: acute	All forms of stretching are contraindicated during the acute stage.	Stretching may aggravate the condition.
Tendinopathies: chronic	Stretching protocols are varied and unproven.	<ul><li>Stretching may help restore tissue elasticity and decrease strain on the musculotendinous junction. Stretching will also help maintain normal range of motion in associated joints.</li><li>Many therapists believe that for Achilles tendinopathies, for example, increased dorsiflexion under load (i.e., active stretch on step) is beneficial because collagen repair is stimulated by reloading.</li><li>Passive stretching of the tendon itself may be useful to stimulate repair but in practice may be difficult to apply. Active stretching places considerable load on tendons, something some therapists believe may be helpful in recovery from these conditions.</li></ul>

Common musculoskeletal condition	General stretching recommendations	Rationale
After surgery	Medical approval should be sought before implementing any stretches. Both patient and therapist need to adhere to any post-surgery advice that has been given.	Stretching immediately after surgery is likely to be detrimental to the natural formation of scar tissue, which is needed for healing. Different surgeons and hospitals are likely to have different rehabilitation protocols.
Acute post-surgical	All forms of stretching are contraindicated during the early stages of healing.	Stretching is an important part of the rehabilitative process, yet if started too soon it could potentially redamage tissues and delay the healing process.
Sub-acute post-surgical	With caution, it is important to begin a gentle stretching programme sooner rather than later.	There is likely to be contracture of soft tissues after surgery. Often there is a period of immobility during which soft tissues may stiffen. Early stretching may help with the realignment of collagen fibres in a manner that means fibrous adhesions are less likely later on. Fibrous adhesions impair normal functioning.
	Where possible, elevate an upper limb or lower limb if this was the part of the body to which there was surgery.	Elevation assists venous and lymphatic drainage and thus helps reduce any swelling that would otherwise impair stretching.
	Stretches should always be within the client's pain-free range, whether active or passive.	Pain could indicate reinjury.
	Encourage gentle active movement of the affected body part.	This facilitates stretching of the surrounding tissues, plus a decrease in swelling, especially in injuries to the foot and ankle where the calf muscle assists in venous and lymphatic drainage.
	When performing active stretches, the client should avoid weight bearing through the limb.	This lessens the likelihood of soft tissue damage in the early stages of repair, when proprioception and balance may be impaired and injured tissues not strong enough to stabilize the joint.

- Look back at the stretching recommendations in table 1.1. This table provides the rationale for the stretches for conditions affecting the lower limb, upper limb and trunk. Apply stretches only if you agree with this rationale.

- With each client, always check whether there are any contraindications to stretching. (See page 22 for a list of contraindications.)

- Confirm that the client consents to treatment.

- If stretching causes pain, stop immediately. Most clients understand and can distinguish the difference between the sensation they experience through the stretching of soft tissues and the sensation of pain. Whether active or passive, stretching should feel slightly uncomfortable but should *never* be painful. Encourage feedback. Monitor your client, and stop any stretches that cause pain. It is your responsibility as a therapist to educate your clients in this respect and help dispel the no-pain-no-gain myth.

- Check that clients following a home-care programme of stretches are doing so safely and that the stretches continue to be safe as the clients' situations are altered. For example, a patient moving from a hospital to more independent living may no longer have someone to supervise his stretching programme. Or a person may move from a living environment that is safe to one that is not (e.g., moving from a home with carpets to one with polished floors; one with a handrail on each side of the stairs to one with only one handrail).

- Check that there are no new or altered contraindications. A client rehabilitating from one condition often suffers another injury. For example, a client may be recovering from a sprained ankle and seem to be doing well, but then she falls because of an imbalance and resprains her ankle or injures her wrist or back. It is important to always check in with your clients so you can modify a stretch or remove it entirely from their programmes.

- If in any doubt about whether or not to use stretching as a treatment intervention, consult with the client's medical practitioner. Get specific approval and guidance.

Finally, it is good to remember that stretching in itself is usually safe. If you follow the guidelines set out in this book and the stretches suggested, it is extremely unlikely that you will cause harm to any of the clients whom you are treating for the conditions included here. At worst your stretching plan could be ineffective; at best it may be useful in helping to meet one of your identified treatment objectives and make a positive contribution to a person's rehabilitation.

Closing Remarks

In this introductory chapter, we have explored the concept of therapeutic stretching, the challenge of designing a stretching protocol for use after injury and the rationale behind the stretches included in this book. In chapter 2 you will find everything you need to help you plan a programme of stretching with your clients.

Quick Questions

1. Define therapeutic stretching.
2. List five other possible treatment interventions besides therapeutic stretching.
3. Describe the difference between a sprain and a strain.
4. List three of the reasons people stretch.
5. From the list of general stretching guidelines, which three are most important to you personally?

Preparing for Stretching

In chapter 1, we examined how therapeutic stretching differs from other forms of stretching and why it is needed. The focus of this chapter is to help you plan a stretching programme by following 10 simple steps:

1. Assess the client.
2. Identify treatment objectives.
3. Choose a stretching method.
4. Set stretching goals.
5. Screen for contraindications.
6. Contemplate the stretching environment.
7. Take measurements.
8. Create a stretching plan.
9. Carry out stretches.
10. Reassess and document findings.

The rest of this chapter discusses these 10 steps.

Step 1: Assess the Client

Whether you are working in the capacity of massage therapist, physical therapist or osteopath, or any other health or fitness professional, you will be familiar with taking a client's case history and will understand the importance of this. The information you gather during this initial consultation serves as your starting point and is likely to contain answers to questions commonly asked by all professionals working with your client. During this consultation it is usual to ask clients to complete a general health questionnaire and to answer questions concerning the history of their condition. This meeting is essential not only to help you gain rapport with your client but also to let you discover any serious illnesses or issues that may affect whether or not you can proceed to treat this client. The form this assessment takes may be governed by a protocol already set within the environment in which you work (such as a hospital or gymnasium) or by the body governing your profession. Whatever the documentation you are using, at the end of the initial consultation you will have identified your client's main problem (prioritizing issues if there are more than one).

Step 2: Identify Treatment Objectives

Next you need to identify the treatment objectives based on this consultation. Examples of treatment objectives include the following:

- To help alleviate pain in the upper trapezius due to muscle tension
- To overcome cramping in the hamstrings of the right thigh
- To improve range of motion in the left knee joint after partial knee replacement surgery
- To help a client adhere to our general stretching programme
- To help a golfer alleviate feelings of stiffness in the lumbar spine

Step 3: Choose a Stretching Method

Once you have identified your treatment objective, your next step might be to choose a stretching method (providing of course that stretching is a useful intervention). There are many different types of stretching. The two main types are active and passive. Active stretches are those a client carries out for herself; passive stretches are those that require a partner, enabling the recipient of the stretch to relax whilst her partner (usually a therapist, trainer or teammate) applies the stretch. Other types of stretching include soft tissue release (STR) and muscle energy technique (MET). If you are new to stretching, it would be helpful to first read chapter 4 (page 43), where these types of stretching are described. Second, take a look at chapters 5, 6 or 7 (depending on whether you need stretching ideas for the lower limb, upper limb or trunk, respectively), and select appropriate stretches from the pathologies listed. These chapters contain examples of both active and passive stretches and are particularly useful for therapists who are new to therapeutic stretching. However, if you believe you need to use STR or MET forms of stretching, refer to *Soft Tissue Release* (J. Johnson, Human Kinetics 2009) and *Facilitated Stretching* (E. McAtee and J. Charland, Human Kinetics 1999).

Step 4: Set Stretching Goals

Once you have identified your treatment objectives and considered which type of stretching might be most appropriate, you need to set stretching goals that you believe will help you and your client meet these objectives. To help you understand how to relate a stretching goal to a treatment objective, each of the five sample treatment objectives in step 2 has been listed in table 2.1 and paired with an appropriate stretching goal. For example, if your treatment objective is to help a client alleviate pain in the upper trapezius due to muscle tension, you might set the goal of performing two different active neck stretches, (A) and (B); providing the client with illustrations of these stretches; and recommending that he perform each stretch twice a day for a minimum of 30 seconds.

Notice that these goals are SMART. That is, they are specific, measurable, achievable, realistic and timely. (See page 27 for ideas on measuring the effectiveness of stretching.) Note also that these goals are examples only. You may have different treatment objectives and different goals. Also, your stretching goals are likely to form part of an overall treatment plan and may not be the only intervention you are using to help meet a particular treatment objective. In the first example, where the objective is to help alleviate tension-induced pain in the upper fibres of the trapezius, it is unlikely that stretching alone will combat this problem. It may be that the client needs to take regular breaks from her workstation (if the maintenance of a static work posture is contributing to her neck pain), apply heat or receive massage as part of her treatment. If you have identified a treatment objective for which stretching is either not appropriate or is not the most beneficial therapeutic intervention, then you would use a different intervention and not do any stretching at all.

Table 2.1 Examples of Therapeutic Goals

Treatment objective	Example of a stretching goal
To help alleviate pain in the upper trapezius due to muscle tension	Client to perform active neck stretches (A) and (B) twice daily, holding each stretch for a minimum of 30 seconds.
To overcome cramping in the hamstrings of the right thigh	Client to perform active hamstring stretch (C) when cramping occurs, maintaining this position until the cramp subsides. Also, client to keep a diary documenting when hamstring cramping occurs, making a note of any activity or inactivity that preceded the event.
To improve range of motion in the left knee joint after partial knee replacement surgery	Client to increase flexion in the left knee by 10 degrees over the next 7 days by performing MET to quadriceps once daily as part of an overall physical therapy programme. MET to be performed as set out in the Basic MET Protocol in chapter 4.
To help a client adhere to our general stretching programme	Client to keep a stretching diary over the next 7 days, placing a tick mark next to each of the stretches on the general hospital stretching programme when the client adopts these positions for 1 minute each.
To help a golfer alleviate feelings of stiffness in the lumbar spine	Over the next 30 days, client to perform stretches (F) and (K) after each game of golf, resting in each stretch position for 2 minutes.

Figures (A), (B), (C), (F) and (K) relate to specific stretches you may have on file, pictures of which you would include in your treatment notes.

Step 5: Screen for Contraindications

Most people benefit from stretching. However, as with all forms of therapy, it is important to identify any clients for whom stretching may be contraindicated or where caution is required. Once you have identified the type of stretching you intend to use and selected any individual stretches, you next need to screen your client for contraindications to these. The following are contraindications to stretching:

- Acute conditions, including recent fracture, ligament sprain, muscle or tendon strain, burns or lacerations
- Inflammatory conditions
- Haematoma
- Vascular disorders of the vertebral artery
- Osteoporosis and patients at risk of fracture
- Malignancy
- Bone or joint limitation (e.g., ankylosing spondylitis; joint fused surgically)
- Acute thrombus or embolism
- Where a muscle contributes to stability in the patient, and to lessen the contracture through stretching would be destabilizing
- When treating a patient where it is not known whether stretching will be beneficial, and medical permission has not been granted
- When stretching could reverse or impair the benefits of another treatment
- Where stretching may compromise the healing process of any condition (e.g., where it might stress a not-yet-healed scar)
- In the inflammatory stages of rheumatoid conditions
- Where the application, either active or passive, causes pain

If you have any doubt about whether stretching may be contraindicated or cautioned, seek the advice of the client's medical practitioner.

Note that a client recovering from a sprained wrist, for example, may still benefit from having other parts of his body stretched even where stretching to the wrist itself is totally contraindicated. In some circumstances stretching is not contraindicated, but it is prudent to exercise some caution. Caution must be used in the following circumstances:

- When passively stretching patients unable to provide feedback about how stretching feels
- When passively stretching clients with fragile skin
- When passively stretching clients where there is high risk of cross infection between therapist and client
- When passively stretching nervous or anxious clients or those for whom there are emotional issues surrounding physical touch

- When passively stretching clients after long-term steroid use
- When prescribing active stretches for patients with balance problems
- When prescribing active stretches to clients who are unable to safely follow simple stretching instructions
- When providing stretches (whether active or passive) for hypermobile patients
- When providing stretches (whether active or passive) for pregnant clients

Almost anyone can receive stretching, and most people will benefit from it. However, there are certain groups of people for whom special consideration is required before implementing a stretching programme. The following sections provide tips to help you modify your stretches so they are safer and more effective when you are working with the elderly, pregnant women and active individuals.

Older Adults

Here are some common physical changes seen in older adults and tips for modifying a stretching programme.

Osteoporosis
Avoid stretches that place excessive stress on bones.

Osteoarthritis
- Avoid stretches that load weight-bearing joints because this may cause pain.
- Stretches to maintain and improve ROM are often beneficial, but remember there may be decreased ROM due to swelling or the formation of osteophytes.
- Useful measurement tools include patient perceptions of the reduction of their joint stiffness and improved quality of life measures.
- Provide stretches that may be done in a seated or lying position, in a chair or bed.
- Provide aids such as a towel.
- When applying passive stretches, it may be necessary to help clients onto and off of a treatment couch or plinth because standing on one leg may be painful. Providing a small stool may help.

Rheumatoid arthritis
- Do no stretches at all during the inflammatory stage.
- All stretching should be pain free during the stretch, in the hours following, and 24 hours after the stretching was performed.
- Remember that joints may fuse, limiting joint ROM.
- Gentle passive stretching may be beneficial, especially where the client is unable to get into the start position for a stretch, but only in the remission period.

Reduction in extensibility of soft tissues
Acknowledge that joint ROM is likely to be reduced in this age group, and modify stretching goals accordingly.

Reduced balance and proprioception

- Minimize the number of stretches that rely on balance.
- Where possible, select stretches that use a low centre of gravity, such as sitting, kneeling or lying.
- For clients stretching independently, always recommend use of a support such as a handrail, table or sink for stability.
- Avoid stretches that require the client to move from lying to standing positions, or vice versa.

Reduced hearing and vision changes

- Keep verbal commands clear and precise.
- Ensure the stretching environment is quiet.
- Demonstrate all stretches, taking your time to reiterate important points.
- Enlarge pictures that you provide as guides for active stretches.

Reduced strength

- MET stretches may be helpful at maintaining or even improving muscle strength.
- Avoid the use of stretches that rely on strength to maintain a stretching position.
- Where the most appropriate stretch is best performed in a standing position, provide a perch stool or chair close by.

Increased medication

Where possible, time stretches to coincide with medication. For example, passive stretches may be more appropriate after medication that is sedative.

Pregnant Women

Here are some common physiological changes seen in pregnant women and tips for modifying a stretching programme.

Loosening of connective tissues

- Avoid taking stretches to their point of maximum resistance.
- Avoid stretches that involve weight bearing through joints that may be in a compromised position.
- Avoid stretches to the hip adductor muscles.
- Avoid stretches that involve excessive flexion or extension of the spine.

Altered balance

- Choose stretches that involve a low centre of gravity, such as those in kneeling or sitting positions.
- In early stages of pregnancy, supine, prone and side-lying positions may be possible provided they are comfortable.

Fatigue in back muscles

Avoid stretches that place additional load on muscles of the back.

Supine hypotension
Avoid stretches in the supine position, especially in late stages of pregnancy.

Active Individuals

Here are some common characteristics of people involved in sport and physical activity and tips for modifying a stretching programme.

There may be increased significance placed on stretching. Stretches may be performed as part of a sporting tradition but may not necessarily be beneficial physiologically.

- Acknowledge the importance these clients place on stretching.
- Respect the use of stretching as part of tradition.
- Be wary of making too many changes too soon to an existing programme of stretches.
- Avoid criticizing the tradition of stretching you believe to be inappropriate.

Regular participation in sporting activity may result in muscle imbalance specific to that sport.

Provide stretches that are sport specific rather than generalized.

An athlete may suffer emotionally when injury prevents training or participation in sport.

- When providing stretches during rehabilitation, acknowledge the impact injury can have on the athlete.
- Identify whether the athlete is demotivated or overly enthusiastic.

Many elite athletes have a good knowledge of stretching. At lower levels of competition, an athlete may be performing inadequate stretches or an inappropriate stretching programme.

- Advice and explanations can be less detailed than those provided for other client groups.
- Do not make assumptions about competency in stretching knowledge. Check in with your client regarding his knowledge of appropriate stretching.

Static stretching may be disadvantageous before a sporting event.

- Avoid sustained static stretching in pre-event situations.
- Use dynamic stretching before sporting events.

Some female athletes may be at risk of osteoporosis.

If in any doubt, avoid stretches that place undue load on vulnerable joints or bones.

Team players often stretch together.

Provide advice and demonstrations of suitable partner stretches.

Often an athlete is under the care of many other professionals.

Commit to working as part of a multidisciplinary team.

Step 6: Contemplate the Stretching Environment

Once you are certain that a client may receive stretching, you need to consider the environment in which the stretches are to be carried out. Just because stretching *can* be performed in a particular environment does not mean this is the most appropriate place for it to be carried out. Parks and open spaces provide ample space to stretch, but not everyone wants to stretch in public. Conversely, some clients may be restricted to a hospital room or ward and have little choice but to stretch within those confines. All environments provide opportunities for stretching. Table 2.2 sets out the advantages and disadvantages associated with each.

Table 2.2 Advantages and Disadvantages of Different Stretching Environments

Environment	Advantages	Disadvantages
Hospital	■ Enables a patient to perform stretches under guidance of a physical therapist ■ Extra equipment is usually available	■ Lack of privacy ■ Lack of space ■ Must coordinate stretching programme with other medical interventions ■ Often patients are on medication that may impair stretching ■ Safety issues (e.g., patients with drips or catheters) ■ Possible cost implication in private hospitals
Home	■ Improved privacy ■ May be carried out at the convenience of the client	■ Stretches are performed unsupervised ■ Requires self-discipline ■ Possible distractions (e.g., family, neighbours, pets, TV, telephone) ■ Some homes lack the necessary space for stretching
Private gym	■ Qualified fitness professionals are on hand for support and guidance ■ Usually there is plenty of space ■ Extra equipment is often available	■ Cost of joining a gym ■ In busy gyms there is sometimes lack of privacy
Park	■ Plenty of space ■ Often there are benches, trees or walls that may be utilized to facilitate stretching ■ Nice environment in summer ■ Fresh air and sunlight ■ Partner stretching can be done here too ■ Could be combined with an outdoor exercise regime	■ Not good for people who feel self-conscious in public (although often private areas can be found) ■ Not so much fun in poor weather or when it is cold

Environment	Advantages	Disadvantages
Office	■ Opportunity to perform stretches daily at work ■ Can be an excuse to get up from a desk and take a break ■ Could be implemented as a group or team programme, thus increasing chances of participation and maintenance of a programme	■ May lack privacy ■ May lack space ■ May be noisy ■ May be distractions (such as telephone calls) ■ Lacks supervision by qualified therapist or fitness professional
Commuting	■ Excellent for alleviating tension of long journeys ■ On car journeys can be a good excuse for the driver to stop and take a break	■ Not suitable for all journeys ■ Lack of privacy ■ Lack of space ■ Type of stretches that may be performed is limited
Therapy (e.g., massage)	■ Can easily be combined with a massage treatment ■ Good opportunity to receive passive stretching ■ Stretches are performed by qualified therapist	■ Cost involved ■ Limited to how often the therapy is performed; therefore not suitable for a programme that needs daily implementation

Step 7: Take Measurements

Next you may want to carry out tests that will later help you measure the effectiveness of your treatment. There are several different ways to measure the effectiveness of a stretching programme. If you are working in a hospital, it may be important to measure and monitor a patient's range of motion in a joint before discharge. Or you might be treating an athlete who wants to achieve a certain degree of flexibility in her hamstring muscles and is interested in measuring this. In most cases, you will need to document your progress, and to do this you will need to take some baseline measurements before and after your treatment intervention (i.e., the stretching), whether or not stretches are being employed passively by you or actively by the client as part of a home-care package you provide.

You can use subjective measures (i.e., where the client reports how he is feeling) or objective measures (i.e., those you observe). Identify first what it is you are trying to measure. Do you want to know whether stretching helps a client feel more relaxed or more flexible or better able to cope with a certain activity? In this case, subjective self-report measures may be appropriate. Or do you need to determine whether stretches have improved the range of motion in a joint? For example, have stretches for the plantar flexors of the ankle joint helped improve range of motion in a client with decreased dorsiflexion? Have stretches for the wrist improved ROM in a client after wrist fracture? In these examples it would be more appropriate to use a goniometer. A goniometer is a simple tool commonly used by physical therapists to measure joint angles. Other objective measures include muscle length tests such as the straight leg raise test and the Thomas test. For detailed information on using a goniometer and the ranges of motion considered normal in human joints, refer to *The Clinical Measurement of Joint Motion*

(W.B. Greene and J.D. Heckman, American Academy of Orthopaedic Surgeons 1993). For traditional descriptions of manually testing muscles, see *Muscles: Testing and Function* (F.P. Kendall, P. Provance, and E.K. McCreary, Lippincott Williams & Wilkins 1993).

The measurement tool you choose depends on your treatment goals and the outcome measures you are seeking. The reasons for stretching that were listed in chapter 1 have been set out as treatment objectives in table 2.3 along with ideas for how each might be measured. Note that this table lists measurement tools that *could* be used, not that *should* be used.

Step 8: Create a Stretching Plan

Now that you have established your treatment objective and set some stretching goals, decided on the type of stretches you want to use and screened your client for contraindications, it is time to formulate your plan. You will also have identified the

Table 2.3   Ideas for Measuring the Effectiveness of Stretching

Treatment objective	Possible measurement tool
To help maintain normal muscle functioning	Self-report measures involving attitudes or feelings, such as an increased ability to perform certain tasks related to muscle function; the self-perceived quality of movement when the muscle is activated
To help alleviate pain due to muscle tension	Self-report measures for pain
To overcome cramping in muscles	Self-report measures relating to the intensity of the pain and the frequency of cramping episodes and how long each episode lasts
To maintain or improve range of motion in a joint	■ Joint range using a goniometer or similar device ■ Change in resistance in muscles or end-feel in a joint ■ Muscle length testing, comparing findings against a norm or with the client's other limb
To facilitate muscle healing	Tissue biopsies (useful in clinical trials but impractical in everyday settings)
To help correct postural imbalances	Photographs before and after stretching
To help minimize the development of scar tissue	Tissue biopsies (useful in clinical trials but impractical in everyday settings)
To influence psychological factors, such as to aid relaxation, maintain or improve motivation or stimulate a sense of well-being	Self-report measures for factors such as level of anxiety, stress or well-being

environment in which the stretches are to be performed, arranged any equipment you need and perhaps carried out some measurements. The final part of your preparation involves expanding your stretching goals, putting them into context by answering some basic questions such as the following:

Who is the plan for?

What is the treatment goal?

What method of measurement is being used?

What type of stretching is being used?

Where are the stretches being performed?

When are the stretches performed?

How are the stretches to be performed?

What is the timescale?

Anything else?

Table 2.4 provides examples of two stretching plans, demonstrating how these questions might be answered.

Table 2.4   Two Sample Stretching Plans

PLAN 1: IN HOSPITAL	
Plan questions	**Plan answers**
Who is the plan for?	70-year-old female recovering from total knee replacement
What is the treatment goal?	To increase right knee flexion from 45 degrees to 90 degrees as per our normal discharge requirement
What method of measurement is being used?	Standard goniometer to measure knee flexion and extension
What type of stretching is being used?	Muscle energy technique to quadriceps following MET protocol; the low-level isometric contraction of the quadriceps muscles will have the added benefit of strengthening the lower limb before discharge
Where are the stretches being performed?	In patient's hospital cubicle
When are the stretches performed?	Twice daily
How are the stretches to be performed?	Patient sitting in high-backed chair, therapist kneeling
What is the timescale?	Discharge planned within 7-10 days
Anything else?	Confirm medical approval before application of the programme; consider use of ice to help reduce swelling before application of the stretch

»continued

»continued

PLAN 2: AT HOME	
Plan questions	**Plan answers**
Who is the plan for?	30-year-old male with stiff low back from long period of bed rest after fracture to right tibia
What is the treatment goal?	To decrease feelings of stiffness in the lumbar spine
What method of measurement is being used?	Self-report measures; stiffness especially noted when client tried to put on shoes and socks and turn taps when in bath
What type of stretching is being used?	Three active stretches for the lumbar spine (W, X, Y)
Where are the stretches being performed?	At home
When are the stretches performed?	Daily
How are the stretches to be performed?	Supine, knee hugging (W) Seated, trunk flexion (X) Standing, pelvic tilting (Y)
What is the timescale?	Until feelings of stiffness decrease
Anything else?	No

Letters in brackets (W, X, Y) refer to illustrations of stretches that would be documented in the client's therapy notes.

Step 9: Carry Out Stretches

Now that you have established your plan, refer back to the general safety guidelines on page 11 in chapter 1, and once you are confident that the stretches you have selected are likely to be both safe and effective, it's time to carry them out.

Step 10: Reassess and Document Findings

As with all forms of therapy, it is useful to document the success (or failure) of a treatment intervention. Was the stretching programme you devised effective at meeting your treatment objectives? If not, why not? Reassess your client, and compare your findings with pre-stretch scores.

Finally, on the basis of your reassessment, decide whether to continue with the stretching programme, revise it or withdraw stretching entirely as a treatment intervention. Usually a client improves as a result of the rehabilitative process, but sometimes a person fails to implement active stretches or his medical condition changes so that stretching is contraindicated. Sometimes a client simply becomes bored of a stretching routine, and it is necessary to introduce new stretches.

Closing Remarks

Hopefully, this chapter has raised your awareness about the variety of elements that need to be taken into consideration when preparing a stretching plan and also given you ideas on treatment objectives, how stretching goals might be set, the advantages and disadvantages of various stretching environments and the sorts of methods that might be used to measure the effectiveness of a stretching programme. In the next part of the book, you will find descriptions of four of the most commonly used forms of stretching along with some of their advantages and disadvantages. Use the material in part II to help inform your decisions about the kinds of stretching programme you select for your clients.

Quick Questions

1. What does SMART stand for with relation to goal setting?
2. List the four types of stretching mentioned in this chapter.
3. When working with elderly patients, why might it be important to provide stretches that are performed in seated or lying positions rather than in the standing position?
4. What is a goniometer?
5. Why is it important to reassess a client after the use of a stretching plan?

PART II

Stretching Methods

There are many ways to stretch soft tissues, and in this part of the book you will find descriptions of some of these. The two most commonly used forms of stretching are those that make up the majority of stretches in part III: active stretching and passive stretching. These two forms of stretching are described in chapter 3, where they are compared and their advantages and disadvantages are identified.

In chapter 4 you will find descriptions of two popular forms of advanced stretching: muscle energy technique (MET) and soft tissue release (STR). Whilst there are few MET and STR stretches included in part III, most of the passive stretches that *are* included form the starting positions for MET stretching. Once you have read the basic MET protocol, you might be able to progress your passive stretches into MET stretches. STR stretching is included as an example of a form of stretching completely different to active, passive or MET, one that is especially useful for incorporating stretching into a massage routine. At the end of chapters 3 and 4 you will again find some quick questions you can use to test your understanding of the material presented here.

Active and Passive Stretching

This chapter begins with a definition of active and passive stretching and then outlines the advantages and disadvantages of each. The two methods are then compared, and tips are provided for therapists wanting to use either stretching method to help rehabilitate clients with the musculoskeletal conditions outlined in chapter 1.

Active and Passive Stretching Definitions, Advantages and Disadvantages

Active stretches are those that a person performs for herself, without the assistance of a therapist or trainer. These are the stretches a person might perform before or after exercise as part of a warm-up or cool-down routine, without assistance from anyone else. They are the kinds of stretches a physical therapist might provide for a patient to do whilst in hospital or at home as part of a rehabilitative programme. The responsibility for carrying out a programme of active stretches rests solely with the person performing it.

The stretches included in an active programme may be static or ballistic. Static stretches are the most safe and involve holding the stretch position for a minimum of around 30 seconds. With this type of stretching the client relaxes into the stretch, allowing his soft tissues to slowly lengthen. Ballistic stretches involve rhythmic kicking or swinging movements where the aim is to increase the degree of stretch with each ballistic movement rather than to hold the stretch position. Relative to other forms of stretching, ballistic stretching is associated with a higher incidence of injury, and whilst it does have its place—notably in sports that require sudden explosive movements such as martial arts—it is not included in this book; ballistic stretching is not appropriate for the rehabilitation of clients recovering from musculoskeletal conditions such as sprains or strains or those needing to combat tight muscles, cramps or stiff joints.

By comparison, passive stretches are those that require the assistance of another person. This second party—usually a fitness professional, physical therapist or sports massage therapist—is responsible for working in conjunction with the client, positioning the client's body in such a way as to facilitate the stretch. A stretching partner may help a client into a stretch position, helping her remain in this position for around 30 seconds. This is the simplest form of passive stretching and is good to learn because it forms the basis of more advanced forms of stretching such as MET.

Bodyworkers have good opportunities to incorporate stretching into a rehabilitative programme. A quick flick through chapters 5, 6 and 7 will reveal that many varieties of stretching positions may be used, whether these are active or passive. So, once you have identified that stretching is likely to help you and your client achieve a particular treatment goal, how do you decide whether to use active stretches or passive stretches or a combination of both? One way is to examine the advantages and disadvantages of each.

An advantage of active stretching is that clients may do it almost anywhere, without having to rely on a therapist being present. The client has complete control over when and where he performs his stretching routine. It can be performed equally well in the privacy of his home or in a hospital environment. It is particularly helpful in the early stages of rehabilitation after injuries such as sprains and strains where passive stretching is contraindicated, or where tissues are particularly stiff and the body weight of the client can help load tissues in such as way as to improve the stretch. One of the disadvantages is that in the absence of a therapist some clients may perform stretches incorrectly. They may either be in the wrong stretching position or fail to hold the stretch for the required amount of time for it to be effective. It can be boring for some clients to maintain a stretching programme, and compliance with such programmes is known to be poor. In some cases active stretching is not suitable. For example, it is not suitable for clients who need supervision for health and safety reasons, and it does not work for those clients who have difficulty getting into or maintaining the stretch position without assistance.

Passive stretching has the advantage of enabling the person being stretched to relax, perhaps facilitating a greater lengthening in soft tissues. It is relatively easy to perform, which may mean the client is more likely to complete a rehabilitative stretching programme than if she were left to her own devices. It can add an element of fun and diversity when used as part of a sporting team's preparation, and although slightly more space is needed than for active stretching, it can be performed almost anywhere. A disadvantage is that the person facilitating the stretch needs to be attuned to the client to avoid overstretching and potentially tearing soft tissues. The client therefore needs to trust his stretching partner and follow the advice given by the therapist or fitness professional with whom he is working, always letting this person know if the passive stretch causes pain. The main disadvantage of passive stretching is that in order for it to be performed, a therapist or trainer needs to be present, and this is not always possible and may incur certain costs.

Now that you have had the opportunity to consider the advantages and disadvantages of these two basic forms of stretching, you might already have some ideas about how you are going to incorporate one or both of them into your rehabilitative programmes, along with the advice or information you might need to give to your clients regarding each. The next two sections outline guidelines for the use of active and passive stretches.

Comparing Active and Passive Stretching

Active stretching

- The client may perform stretches on her own with no need for a stretching partner.
- Active stretching doesn't cost anything.

- This places the responsibility for stretching with the client, engaging the client with his own rehabilitation.

- With active stretching the client needs to be motivated in order to carry out the programme.
- Active stretching can help add variety to a home exercise routine and thus keep clients engaged and motivated in the self-management of a condition.
- The possibility for error is high because some clients misunderstand how to perform stretches.
- Only a small selection of stretches may be performed each week because providing a client with too many stretches risks non-compliance with the programme.
- Certain clients will benefit more from receiving passive stretching, especially where their conditions prevent them from getting into a comfortable or safe stretching position.
- It is difficult for clients to know how to modify stretches where necessary unless they are themselves a therapist.
- Self-reporting measures can be used to determine the effectiveness of stretches, but a therapist is required where objective measurement is needed.
- The effort of getting into and maintaining a stretch position may mean some clients find it harder to relax, and this may prevent them from enjoying the full benefit of the stretch.

Passive stretching

- The therapist or stretching partner needs to be present.

- There is often a cost involved (i.e., payment to a therapist, fitness professional or coach).

- This places the responsibility for stretching with the therapist rather than with the client, although in most cases the client is required to participate by providing feedback.
- This does not rely on the client's being motivated to carry out a stretching programme.
- Passive stretching can be used to add variety to a massage routine because it is easily incorporated into a massage sequence.
- The likelihood for errors is decreased because most therapists will apply stretches correctly.
- It is likely that a considerable number of stretches could be performed should these be required.

- Passive stretches are useful in treating clients who are unable to get into certain stretching positions.

- The therapist can easily modify stretches should this be necessary.

- Having a therapist present means objective measures can easily be used to record the effectiveness of stretching.
- Clients can fully relax as they receive passive stretching because the therapist helps move limbs into position and places gentle tension on soft tissues.

Guidelines for Providing
an Active Stretching Programme

If you have chosen to provide your client with active stretches, the following guidelines may be helpful:

- Select only one or two easy stretches to start with. Many people do not adhere to the advice given to them by therapists, so it is best to keep things simple. The easier a stretching programme appears to the client, the more likely she will adhere to it.

- By contrast, highly motivated clients may need a greater number of stretches in order to stay engaged and in a positive frame of mind, especially if they are keen to return to physical activity.

- Unless the client is already competent with stretching, demonstrate the stretch you want him to do.

- Ask the client to perform the stretch. Observe how she does it, and make any necessary adjustments. For example, if she seems unstable performing a stretch you have chosen in a standing position, consider using a seated stretch as an alternative.

- Provide the client with an illustration of each stretch. Clearly document how to do the stretch, when to do it and for how long to hold the stretch position. Be specific. For example, "Perform stretch A once each morning on both left and right legs and once each afternoon on both left and right legs, holding each stretch for 45 seconds."

- Provide safety advice. For example, be sure a client understands what "within your pain-free range" means. This is particularly important when providing stretches for clients to do in the sub-acute stages of injury.

- Actively discourage the no-pain-no-gain approach.

- Modify stretches where necessary, and compromise where necessary. For example, stretching the calf muscles might be more effective when the client is in bare feet, but it may be inconvenient for an elderly client to remove and put on footwear.

- When you next see your client, ask him to show you how he has been doing the stretches. Has he been doing them correctly? Were there any problems? Did he find the stretches beneficial? Document your findings.

- Provide a stretching diary so the client can document progress for herself. An example of a stretching diary is provided on page 39. This is a useful way for a patient to record which stretches she has performed simply by placing a tick mark next to each day of the week. Including a comments box is useful so the client can record how she felt; detail any observed improvements (e.g., decreased pain), improved ability (e.g., being able to reach behind her back to do up a bra) or difficulties encountered (e.g., losing balance whilst stretching, difficulty getting into or out of a stretching position); and document anything else she thinks might be relevant.

SIMPLE STRETCHING DIARY

	Mon	Tue	Wed	Thu	Fri	Sat	Sun

Stretch A
Perform once per day, holding
the end position for 45 seconds

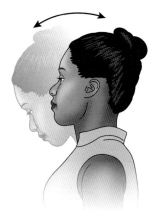

Stretch B
Perform once per day (each
side), holding the stretch position for 45 seconds

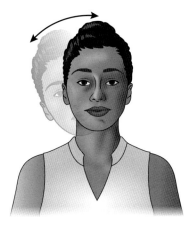

Comments

From J. Johnson, 2012, *Therapeutic stretching* (Champaign, IL: Human Kinetics).

- Vary the stretches you provide for clients every three or four days or weekly in order to increase the likelihood of adherence.

- Always check to see whether the stretches you have provided are meeting your treatment goals.

Guidelines for Applying Passive Stretches

If you wish to use passive stretches, whether in conjunction with an active stretching programme or as a stand-alone stretching programme, you can help ensure your work is both effective and safe by adhering to these basic guidelines:

- Always start with your client in a comfortable position.

- Explain what it is you are going to do, and give the client clear instructions for anything *he* needs to do.

- Encourage the client to breathe normally. Some clients have a tendency to hold their breath in anticipation of being stretched by another person. Whilst the use of breathing can enhance stretching, this is something that requires practice and should be adopted only after you and the client have gained each other's trust. Until then, discourage your clients from holding their breath when they are being stretched.

- Encourage the client to let you know if she experiences any discomfort or pain, and if she does, stop the stretch immediately. You are totally reliant on the client's reporting how she is feeling. Of course, you may sense an increase in muscle tension, something that occurs naturally when we are in pain, but you should not be stretching so vigorously or with such force as to elicit an increase in tension in this manner.

- Since you will need to hold the client's limbs in order to facilitate the stretch, be sensitive about where you position your hands. For example, be careful not to place your hands too high on the inner thigh or too close to the breasts.

- Take the limb being stretched to a point where the client feels mild resistance. Hold this position. Only once the tension in tissues has eased should you ease the limb further into the stretch position, holding it as soon as you sense a barrier to the stretch. Proceed in this manner even when working with clients reporting extreme stiffness.

- Take your time. When your aim is to help a client experience a good stretch and an improvement in joint range, it can be frustrating when progress seems slow. Most therapists want to gain as much improvement as possible, especially if they have limited time or will not have an opportunity to work with that particular client for some days. However, do not be tempted to rush your stretching. It is better to stretch little and often than to try to force tissues to lengthen.

- Follow the simple passive stretching protocol set out here:
  1. Assuming there are no contraindications and with the client in a comfortable position, take the tissues being stretched to their natural point of resistance, using your client to guide you on where this point is.

2. Hold the tissues in this position for a minimum of 30 seconds, encouraging the client to breathe normally.

3. Either help the client out of the stretch position or gently increase the stretch, repeating steps 1 and 2.

Closing Remarks

If you have identified what form of stretching you think is most appropriate for your client, turn to the relevant chapter in part III for descriptions of many stretches for use on different parts of the body. For example, if you are treating a client with a lower limb problem, turn to chapter 5; for those clients needing upper limb stretches, look at chapter 6; and when treating clients with neck or back problems, refer to chapter 7. At the start of each chapter, you will find a table showing where to locate active and passive stretches within that chapter for all the relevant musculoskeletal conditions listed in chapter 1. Additionally, you might like to read chapter 4, which describes two commonly used forms of advanced stretching, STR and MET.

Quick Questions

1. Define active stretching.
2. Define passive stretching.
3. When working with a client for the first time, why do you think it is important to provide only one or two easy stretches if you are assigning active stretching?
4. Both active and passive stretches should be held for a minimum length of how many seconds?
5. When applying a passive stretch to the limb of a client, how do you know to which point to take the limb before holding the stretch position?

Advanced Forms of Stretching

The stretches provided in part III of this book are predominantly active and passive stretches. It is nevertheless advisable to consider two advanced forms of stretching, muscle energy technique (MET) and soft tissue release (STR) because these are both useful when treating some of the musculoskeletal conditions discussed in this text. Very basically, MET is helpful when working with clients in the early stages of rehabilitation after injury, whilst STR might be more appropriate for clients with chronically tight muscles. The purpose of this chapter is not to provide detailed information on carrying out MET and STR but to highlight that there are other very useful techniques you might wish to explore once you are competent in the use of active and passive stretching. The chapter provides an overview of two of these.

Muscle Energy Technique

Popularly known simply as MET, muscle energy technique is a form of stretching commonly used by sports massage therapists, sports therapists, osteopaths and some physiotherapists, chiropractors and fitness professionals. There is no standardized definition of this technique, which involves the active contraction of a muscle by the client against a resistive force provided by a second party (i.e., the therapist). Originating as an osteopathic technique in the late 1950s and early 1960s, there are today numerous variations and applications of this method of stretching.

MET is believed to be particularly helpful in lengthening postural muscles, which are prone to shortening. Theoretically, the active contraction performed by the client against the resistance produced by the therapist is an isometric contraction and may therefore be helpful in strengthening muscles. Also, contraction of one muscle group decreases tone in the opposing muscle group, and MET may therefore be beneficial in helping to overcome cramping. There is some debate about the degree of force a client should use when contracting a muscle before it is stretched, although low levels of contraction are advocated, certainly no more than 25 percent of the client's maximum force capacity. This is especially important should the technique be used in early stages of rehabilitation after injury, when levels as low as 5 percent may be the most appropriate. MET is sometimes used with a pulsing motion (known as *pulsed MET*), which advocates claim helps reduces localized oedema. MET is therefore used in the following circumstances:

- To stretch muscles, especially those considered to be postural rather than phasic
- To strengthen muscles
- To relax muscles, especially useful for treating cramping muscles
- To help regain correct muscle function
- To reduce localized oedema

A disadvantage of this technique is that it may be applied in many ways, and training is required to learn how and when to use each. For further information, please see *Muscle Energy Techniques* (L. Chaitow, Churchill Livingstone 2001), where eight variations on the basic MET technique are described, along with information on how and when they might be used, and on which the basic MET protocol described here is based. *Facilitated Stretching* (E. McAtee and J. Charland, Human Kinetics 1999) is also a good source of starting positions for performing MET stretches.

Basic MET Protocol

A basic MET protocol is as follows:

1. Position the client so that both you and he are comfortable. Take the muscle to be stretched to a resistance *barrier*, that point where both you and the client can feel an increase in the resistance of the client's tissues to further elongation. This barrier is the point at which you will start to stretch. Tell the client to let you know as soon as you reach this barrier, a point where he may feel an ever so slight stretch. This entire procedure should be pain free.

2. Ask the client to contract his muscle (i.e., the one in which he feels the mild stretch) using a maximum of 25 percent of his muscle force, whilst you resist this contraction. Maintain the body part that is being stretched in a static position so the effect is an isometric contraction of the muscle you are about to stretch. It is important that it is the client who sets the level of contraction against which you resist, not the other way around. That is, clients should never be resisting *your* force; you should be resisting *theirs*. Remember, too, that when used as part of rehabilitation, clients should be instructed to use very low levels of contraction, perhaps as low as 5 percent of their maximal force.

3. After about 10 seconds ask the client to relax, and within the next 3 to 5 seconds, gently ease the body part further into the stretch so you find a new barrier position. Maintain this position for a few seconds before repeating the procedure up to two more times.

You may meet therapists who ask a client to contract a muscle for more than 10 seconds, or who wait a couple of seconds before performing the stretch; many hold the client's limb in the final stretch position for some time, encouraging a gentle relaxation of soft tissues. There are many variants on MET stretching, and I encourage you to experiment to discover what works for you.

Getting Started With MET

One of the reasons for including a brief description of MET is that the examples of passive stretches provided in chapters 5, 6 and 7 are all starting positions from which to apply the basic MET protocol described here. For example, if you wanted to apply this basic MET to the calf using this protocol, you would follow these steps:

1. Start with your client in either of the passive stretch positions shown here.
2. Ask your client to use 25 percent of her force to push her toes into your thigh *(a)* or hand *(b)*, plantar flexing her ankles and isometrically contracting her calf muscles.
3. Resist this contraction for 10 seconds. Then, once the client relaxes, gently dorsiflex her foot and ankle within the next 3 to 5 seconds to reach a new resistance barrier.

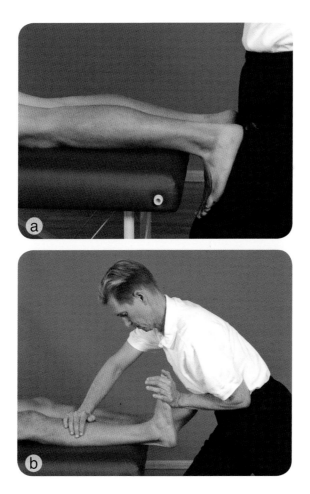

Soft Tissue Release

Soft tissue release is quite different from MET. This form of stretching involves first shortening (rather than lengthening) the muscle to be stretched, then 'locking' a passively shortened muscle close to or on its origin before stretching the muscle, maintaining this lock as the muscle is passively lengthened. Placing these locks closer and closer to the distal insertion point of the muscle results in a decreased amount of tissue that is able to lengthen with each movement, and the result is to localize the stretch to a particular area of muscle, something that may be advantageous when working with clients with chronically tight muscles.

The advantages of STR are as follows:

- Pressure and stretch are believed to facilitate a lengthening of soft tissues and an increase in ROM.
- It may be performed either actively or passively (although not all STR stretches can be performed actively).
- When performed actively, the only equipment required is a tennis ball.
- It can easily be incorporated into a massage sequence (and may also be performed through clothing), so it may be useful where massage is indicated as part of a client's rehabilitation or maintenance programme.
- It may be used to help deactivate trigger points (where the 'lock' is placed over the trigger point).

Following are the disadvantages of STR:

- Therapists need to learn the technique, which can take several forms.
- It cannot be used on all clients (e.g., those who bruise easily or have fragile skin).
- It may result in soreness similar to DOMS in some clients if used too vigorously.

Basic STR Protocol

A basic STR protocol follows:

1. Shorten the muscle that is to be stretched. This may be done actively or passively.
2. Choose a point close to the muscle's origin, and fix the tissues you want to stretch by using your thumbs, fists, forearm or elbow. (Different fixes, or 'locks,' have different effects.) Avoid pressing into joints.
3. Whilst maintaining this lock, actively or passively stretch this muscle.

To see how this might work in practice, please see the next section.

Getting Started With STR

Using the calf muscle again as an example will help you compare this technique with MET.

1. Shorten the calf muscle. In the case of the calf, if you allow your client's foot and ankle to rest off the couch as shown in *a*, the ankle falls naturally into plantar flexion, and the calf muscle is in a shortened position.

2. Lock the calf close to its origin, avoiding the knee joint (*b*).

3. Whilst maintaining this lock, gently use your thigh to stretch the tissues of the calf (*c*).

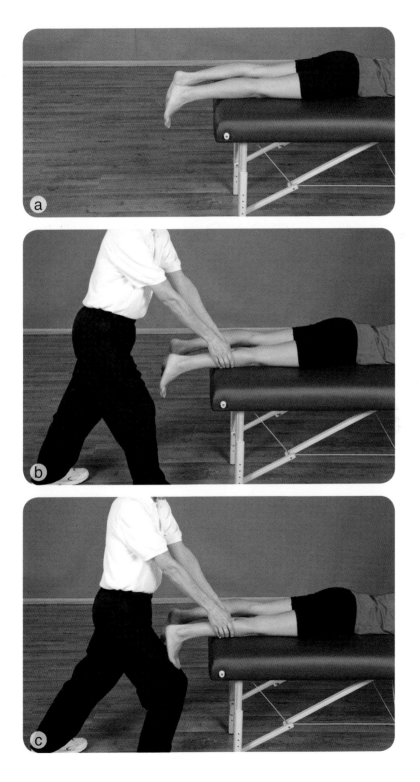

STR is a useful form of stretching when a client cannot take a joint through its full range (e.g., because of injury) or when working with hypermobile clients, where taking a stretch to the client's end-of-joint range may not be desirable. It is also valuable in targeting areas of fibrotic tissue within muscles that would otherwise not be stretched with gross active stretching. For further information, please see *Soft Tissue Release* (J. Johnson, Human Kinetics 2009).

Closing Remarks

You have now been introduced to two other forms of stretching and learned that all the passive stretches in part III serve as the starting positions from which to employ MET stretches, should you wish to follow the simple MET protocol set out here. It is good to remember, however, that as with all forms of stretching, much research is still needed to establish the most effective stretching protocols for both MET and STR.

Quick Questions

1. How much force do you instruct your client to use when actively contracting a muscle before an MET stretch?
2. If you wanted to use the descriptions and photographs in this book as a starting position for MET stretches, would you select the active stretches or the passive stretches?
3. How is STR different from MET?
4. How might you 'lock' tissues when performing STR?
5. List three useful books for finding detailed information on MET and STR.

Implementing Your Stretches

This part of the book is where you will find photos and descriptions of active and passive stretches to use when treating clients with the musculoskeletal conditions listed in chapter 1. Part III has three chapters: chapter 5 (Stretching the Lower Limb), chapter 6 (Stretching the Upper Limb) and chapter 7 (Stretching the Trunk). Each chapter begins with a table listing the conditions for which stretches are provided, grouping these according to whether they are active or passive. For consistency, active stretches always appear first. This does not mean they should always be used first, although when treating clients with sub-acute injuries, the active stretches are most safe.

Stretches have been selected on the basis of their appropriateness and usefulness and to provide you with ideas about the variety of stretches that may be effective. By reading these chapters you should feel inspired to provide clients with active stretches for use as part of their home-care package as well as encouraged to implement some passive stretches as part of your treatment. As you find opportunities to implement the stretches provided here, you will no doubt develop preferences. It is likely that some of these stretches may appeal to you, whilst others may not. Adapt them to suit your needs, and invent others you believe may be more appropriate to the needs of your clients.

Stretching the Lower Limb

Within this chapter are 57 stretches (33 active and 24 passive) for treating conditions commonly affecting the lower limb. Table 5.1 shows which stretches are provided. Here you will find stretches that may help with the rehabilitation of clients with injuries, such as a sprained ankle or a groin strain, as well as more long-term conditions, such as chronic calf and hamstring tightness. Information is also provided on the use of stretching after more serious conditions such as a fractured ankle and after surgery to the knee.

Note: The stretches listed in this table for each pathology are not the *only* stretches that could or should be used. Within each section you will often find tips for modifying a stretch or recommendations to include stretches shown in other parts of this chapter. Additional useful stretches for each pathology are shown in *italics* within table 5.1. The numbers in the table (e.g., 5.1, 5.2) refer to the figure numbers that illustrate the stretch.

Table 5.1 Stretches for the Lower Limb

	Active	Passive
FOOT AND ANKLE		
Ankle sprain: acute	Not recommended	Not recommended
Ankle sprain: sub-acute	5.1, page 54 5.2, page 55 *5.17, page 62*	Not recommended
Achilles tendinopathies: acute	Not recommended	Not recommended
Achilles tendinopathies: sub-acute or chronic	5.3, page 56 5.4, page 56	5.5, page 57 5.6, page 57 *5.14, page 61*
Ankle fracture: acute	Not recommended	Not recommended

»continued

»continued

	Active	Passive
FOOT AND ANKLE		
Ankle fracture: sub-acute	With medical approval, *treat as for a sub-acute ankle sprain* *5.1, page 54* *5.2, page 55* *5.17, page 62*	Not recommended
Stiff ankle	5.7, page 59 5.8, page 59 5.9, page 59 5.10, page 60 5.11, page 60 5.12, page 60 5.13, page 61 *5.3, page 56* *5.4, page 56*	5.14, page 61 5.15, page 61 5.16, page 61 *5.5, page 57* *5.6, page 57* *5.20, page 62*
Plantar fasciitis	5.17, page 62 5.18, page 62 5.19, page 62 *5.7, page 59* *5.8, page 59* *5.10, page 60* *5.11, page 60* *5.12, page 60*	5.20, page 62 *5.5, page 57* *5.6, page 57*
KNEE AND LEG		
Calf muscle strains: acute	Not recommended	Not recommended
Calf muscle strains: sub-acute	Treat as for sub-acute ankle sprain *5.7, page 59* *5.11, page 60* *5.12, page 60*	Not recommended
Shin splints	*5.9, page 59*	5.21, page 64 5.22, page 64
Tight calf muscles	*5.11, page 60* *5.12, page 60* *5.3, page 56* *5.4, page 56*	5.23, page 65 *5.5, page 57* *5.6, page 57* *5.14, page 61*
Cramp in the calf	*5.7, page 59* *5.3, page 56* *5.8, page 59* *5.10, page 60* *5.11, page 60* *5.12, page 60*	*5.5, page 57* *5.6, page 57* *5.14, page 61*
Osteoarthritis in the knee	5.24, page 67 Lower limb stretches in water are also helpful	5.25, page 67 *5.24, page 67*

	Active	Passive
KNEE AND LEG		
After knee surgery	With medical approval, 5.26, page 68 *5.24, page 67*	5.27, page 68
HIP AND THIGH		
Hamstring strain: acute	Not recommended	Not recommended
Hamstring strain: sub-acute	*5.7, page 59* *5.10, page 60* *5.26, page 68*	Not recommended
Tight hamstrings	5.28, page 70 5.29, page 71 5.30, page 71 5.31, page 71 *5.7, page 59* *5.10, page 60* *5.26, page 68* *5.11, page 60*	5.32, page 72 5.33, page 72 5.34, page 72
Hamstring cramp	*5.3, page 56* *5.7, page 59* *5.10, page 60* *5.11, page 60* *5.12, page 60*	5.35, page 73 5.36, page 74
Groin strain: acute	Not recommended	Not recommended
Groin strain: sub-acute	5.37, page 75 5.38, page 75 5.39, page 75	Not recommended
Tight adductors	5.40, page 76 5.41, page 76 *5.37, page 75* *5.38, page 75* *5.39, page 75*	5.42, page 77 5.43, page 77
Tight quadriceps	5.44, page 78 5.45, page 78	5.46, page 79 5.47, page 79
Tight hip flexors	5.48, page 80 5.49, page 80 5.50, page 81	5.51, page 81 5.52, page 81
Iliotibial band friction syndrome (runner's knee)	5.53, page 82 *5.55, page 83* *5.56, page 83*	5.54, page 82 *5.57, page 84*
Piriformis syndrome	5.55, page 83 5.56, page 83	5.57, page 84

Ankle Sprains

An ankle sprain is the wrenching and tearing of ligaments on either the lateral or medial side of the ankle joint, sometimes with damage to the anterior of the joint capsule. The most common form of sprain is an inversion sprain, where the lateral ligaments are damaged. Less common is an eversion sprain where the strong deltoid ligament on the medial side of the ankle is torn. In serious inversion sprains there may be an avulsion fracture to the fifth metatarsal as the fibularis brevis muscle is wrenched from its insertion. With severe eversion sprains, damage to the distal end of the fibula sometimes occurs when sharp eversion of the foot crushes or snaps that end of the bone.

Acute

All forms of stretching are contraindicated for acute ankle sprains.

Sub-Acute

With caution, it is important to begin a gentle stretching programme sooner rather than later as this may help realign collagen fibres in such a way that fibrous adhesions are less likely to occur. However, for safety reasons, stretching should be active only, not weight bearing and well within a client's pain-free range.

Active stretches

Figure 5.1 shows the position most beneficial for the rehabilitation of ankle sprains and in which active movements should be performed. Figure 5.2 shows the four movements of the ankle (dorsiflexion, plantar flexion, eversion and inversion) that need to be restored.

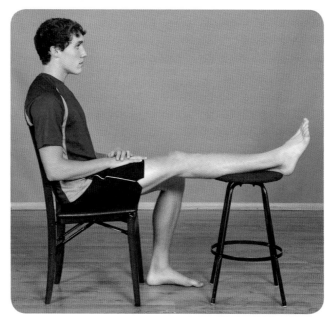

Figure 5.1

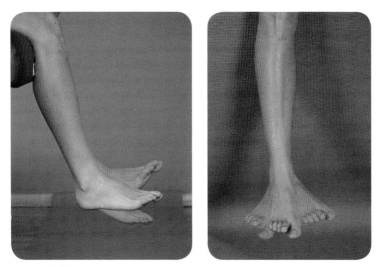

Figure 5.2

The aim of your treatment might be to help the client maintain (and later improve) range of motion in the ankle. Instruct your client in performing gentle dorsiflexion and plantar flexion with the foot elevated as shown in figure 5.1, stressing that this should be within a pain-free range. Later, introduce the movements of eversion and inversion. Dorsiflexion and plantar flexion are used first because the ankle naturally falls into plantar flexion at rest; if the foot is allowed to remain in this position, it will lead to stiffening of the posterior ankle joint and shortening of muscles in the posterior compartment of the leg. Dorsiflexion and plantar flexion are also the easiest ankle movements. Movements of eversion and inversion are harder for most clients to perform, yet they are important to include at some stage of the rehabilitative process because they will help restore range of motion in the joint.

TIP It is important to include stretches to the toes, especially of the flexor muscles (such as in figure 5.17), because the long tendons of these muscles cross the ankle joint and therefore affect ankle ROM.

Once the injury is healed, the client may progress to gentle stretches of the calf (see figures 5.8 and 5.9). Where stretching is not included as part of the rehabilitation programme, the client may experience a stiffening of the ankle joint as soft tissues shorten and adhere to one another.

Achilles Tendinopathies

Unlike the treatment of an ankle sprain, where weight bearing is to be avoided, here it may be safe for sub-acute and chronic tendinopathies and is possibly advantageous as this tendon can withstand remarkably high forces.

Acute

Overuse injuries may be deemed acute if there is inflammation present or if the condition is highly painful. Both active and passive stretches are contraindicated in the acute stage.

Sub-Acute

This stage differs from the acute stage in that both pain and inflammation (if there is any) have subsided, yet the condition persists. The injury is often aggravated by repetitive movement and may therefore limit exercise.

Active stretches

Figure 5.3 shows a useful stretch that is easy to perform daily on a step or stair, using a handrail for support. This position results in eccentric loading of the calf muscles, thought by some therapists to be beneficial.

A squatting soleus stretch (figure 5.4) is also useful and utilizes body weight to help stretch this relatively tough tendon at the same time as the soleus.

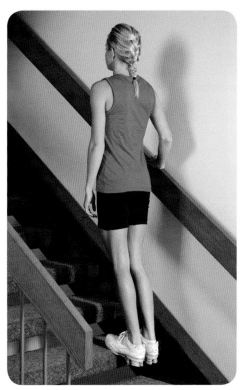

Figure 5.3

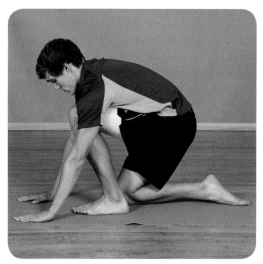

Figure 5.4

Passive stretches

Passive stretches to the gastrocnemius (figure 5.5) and soleus (figure 5.6) in the prone position are effective ways to stretch this strong tendon. Notice that in figure 5.5 the therapist is using the thigh to increase dorsiflexion at the ankle, an action that requires considerable force when using your hand. The stretch shown in figure 5.6 increases the stretch to the soleus muscle but may not be appropriate for clients who are unable to lie prone or for those who have problems with the knee on the side being stretched (as you can see, this particular stretch puts quite a lot of pressure on the knee).

Another stretch that may be helpful is to passively dorsiflex the ankle in the supine position (see figure 5.14). However, these stretches can be less effective for strong, physically active people because the force required to promote the stretch is more difficult to apply with the client in the prone position.

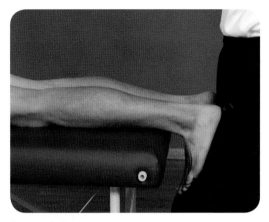

Figure 5.5

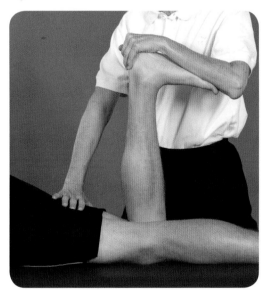

Figure 5.6

Ankle Fracture

An ankle fracture is an acute injury, usually of traumatic nature, accompanied by immediate pain and swelling. The distal ends of the tibia and fibula may be broken, or the talus bone of the ankle. There is usually damage to ligaments of the joint.

Acute

Stretching is contraindicated in the acute stage of an ankle fracture.

Sub-Acute

In the sub-acute stage, pain and swelling are reduced but the ankle is far from being healed, so much caution is required.

Active stretches

Gentle active movements to maintain and improve range of motion may be helpful provided there are no complications and you have medical approval. It is not always possible to perform movements if the ankle is immobilized (e.g., in a cast or brace). However, if movements *are* possible, treat as for a sub-acute ankle sprain (page 54). Advise the client to perform active ROM stretches (see figure 5.2) and to avoid weight-bearing stretches. Remember that immobilization of the ankle will result in decreased mobility in bones of the foot and toes, so suggesting stretches such as figure 5.17 may be useful.

TIP Even when patients have been given medical approval to carry out gentle movements of the ankle, they are often fearful of doing this, perhaps believing it will result in reinjury. Once the fracture is healed, refer to the next section if you need ideas for stretches to help combat ankle stiffness.

Passive stretches

Passive stretches are not recommended for ankle fractures.

Stiff Ankle

Many people suffer from stiff ankles. This condition may result from a sedentary lifestyle or direct immobilization of the lower limb due to surgery. Sometimes clients complain of stiffness resulting from a previous injury where there was little or no intervention; function has been restored, but there remain limitations in range of motion.

Active stretches

Active stretches are useful because the client may incorporate body weight to facilitate a stretch in tissues. For clients with impaired balance or who are unable to bear weight through their lower limbs, gentle dorsiflexion helps stretch the calf (figure 5.7) and soleus (figure 5.8), whilst plantar flexion (figure 5.9) helps stretch the tibialis anterior and the anterior of the ankle joint. Together these stretches help maintain range of motion at the ankle joint.

Note that in figure 5.7 the client is also stretching the tissues of the posterior thigh, including the hamstrings. This position may be uncomfortable for elderly or sedentary clients, in which case dorsiflexion is simply performed with the client seated in a chair. One of the advantages of the stretch in figure 5.7 is that it engages the muscles of dorsiflexion and thus inhibits the plantar flexors that relax and stretch.

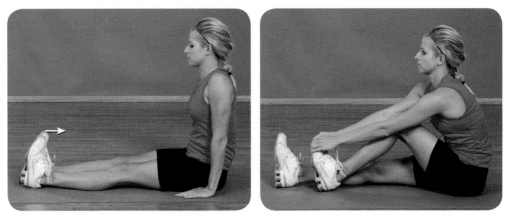

Figure 5.7   Figure 5.8

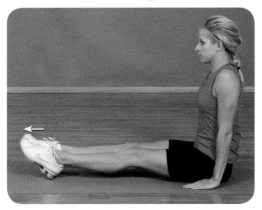

Figure 5.9

Some clients are unable to reach their toes as in figure 5.8 (e.g., pregnant women, overweight people, people with very tight hamstrings or stiff low backs). Using a towel hooked around the toes (figure 5.10) is a helpful alternative.

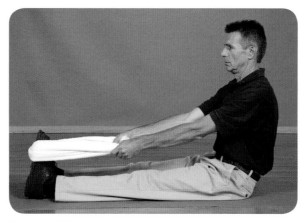

Figure 5.10

Figures 5.11 and 5.12 show standing calf stretches. Slight flexion in the knee joint when performing the stretch increases the stretch to the soleus muscle. Clients who find this stretch easy can try the stretches shown in figures 5.3 and 5.4, which place greater tension on the soleus and Achilles tendon.

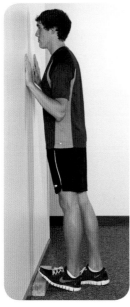
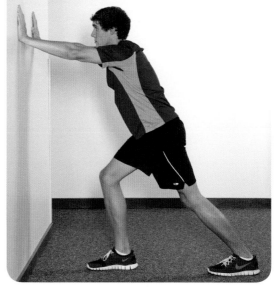

Figure 5.11   Figure 5.12

Placing a towel beneath the lateral side of the foot (figure 5.13) and simply standing in this position helps increase the movement of eversion (by stretching the invertor muscles).

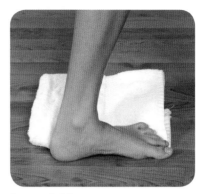

Passive stretches

Passive stretches are useful where a client has not been weight bearing for a period of time and may have lost his sense of balance. Dorsiflexion in the supine position (figure 5.14) and gentle plantar flexion (figure 5.15) are helpful, but remember that the ankle naturally falls into plantar flexion at rest, and it is important not to overstretch the soft tissues of the anterior aspect of this joint when using this position.

Figure 5.13

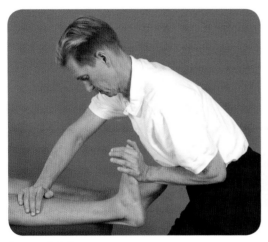

Figure 5.14

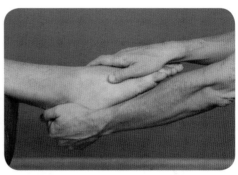

Figure 5.15

TIP When applying either of these stretches, it is often easier if you position the client's foot so it rests just off the treatment couch.

A third useful passive stretch is best performed with the client side-lying. Use a small towel, folded to form a pad that is a little less thick than what is shown in figure 5.16.

Also use the passive stretches illustrated in figures 5.5, 5.6 and 5.20.

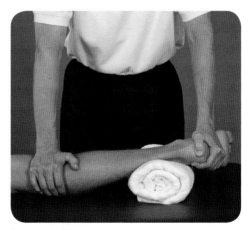

Figure 5.16

Plantar Fasciitis

Microtears in the plantar fascia, popularly misconceived as inflammation and termed plantar fasci*itis*, are extremely painful. The plantar fascia is consistent with the fascia of the calf via the calcaneus, and stretching the tissues of one (i.e., of the foot or of the calf) is likely to improve extensibility in tissues of the other area. Therefore it is always useful to include calf stretches, both active and passive, when treating this condition (see, for example, figures 5.7, 5.8, 5.10, 5.11 and 5.12).

Active stretches

Figures 5.17 and 5.18 illustrate two useful active stretches for the plantar fascia. In figure 5.18, the client has the benefit of being able to use body weight to help facilitate the stretch, but for some clients and in acute stages of the condition, this may be too uncomfortable. A third form of active stretching is for the client to slowly roll the foot over a hard ball such as a golf ball (figure 5.19). This stretches small sections of the fascia, which may have an overall beneficial effect. If you decide to recommend this stretch, make sure the client performs it whilst sitting and does not attempt to stand on the golf ball, but gently rolls the foot over it.

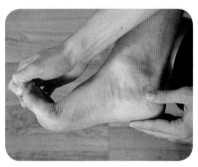

Figure 5.17

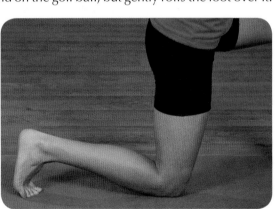

Figure 5.18

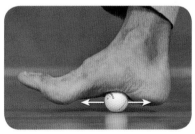

Figure 5.19

Passive stretches

The plantar fascia covers part of the sole of the foot, and stretching the toes into extension, as in figure 5.20, will tension this fascia. Massaging the sole of the foot, using your fingers to spread and stretch the soft tissues of the metatarsal heads, is also helpful providing it is not painful. Stretches in figures 5.5 and 5.6 will help stretch tissues of the calf, which can in turn alleviate discomfort in the plantar fascia.

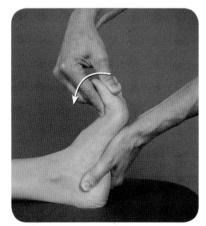

Figure 5.20

Calf Muscle Strains

Calf muscle strains are tears in muscle fibres of the calf and may involve the gastrocnemius, soleus, or both. Strains vary in severity from a few fibres being torn to complete rupture. Localized pain and swelling increase with the severity of the tear, as does the ability to actively plantar flex. Scar tissue is laid down as part of the healing process, the quantity of which depends on the severity of the injury and the quality of rehabilitation the client receives. Large amounts of scar tissue may impair function.

Acute

Even where a strain is believed to be mild, all forms of stretching should be avoided in the acute stages of injury, during which time it is important for tissues to begin their repair process.

Sub-Acute

In the sub-acute stage, pain, swelling and inflammation have subsided. It is wise to be cautious in recommending stretches during this stage because tissues are not yet healed and overzealous stretching could result in reinjury to the muscle, delaying the healing process.

Active stretches

With care, active stretches may be used providing the client remains within a pain-free range. Dorsiflexion of the ankle in a non-weight-bearing position, either seated on a chair or with the legs extended as in figure 5.7, is a good starting stretch. Towards the end of the healing process, and should the client believe the calf is particularly tight, progression to standing calf stretches such as figures 5.11 and 5.12 is recommended. Remember, with calf strains, pain subsides before healing is complete, and clients should be encouraged to stop if any of the stretches cause pain.

Passive stretches

Passive stretching is not recommended for calf muscle strains.

Shin Splints

Shin splints is a generic term used to describe pain on the anterior leg, commonly the result of overuse activities such as running.

Active stretches

A simple active stretch is to point the toes, thus plantar flexing the foot and stretching the tibialis anterior (as in figure 5.9).

Passive stretches

Soft tissue release is helpful in addressing tension in the tissues of the anterior leg. Start by passively shortening the muscle. Next, apply gentle pressure to the muscle (figure 5.21), close to its origin. Maintaining this pressure, lengthen the muscle in question by either passively or actively plantar flexing the ankle (figure 5.22). When you have done this, select a different spot on the muscle, perhaps distal to where you first applied pressure, and repeat the process of first shortening the muscle, then applying pressure and maintaining this pressure whilst plantar flexing the ankle.

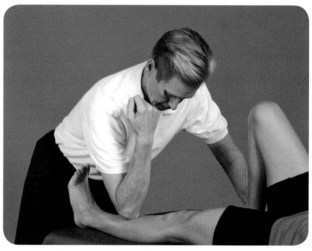

Figure 5.21

Note that in this example, a therapist experienced in the use of STR is using the elbow to gently compress the tibialis anterior. If you are unfamiliar with this technique, it is better to start by gently fixing or locking the muscle using your thumbs to avoid potentially bruising the tissues covering the shin.

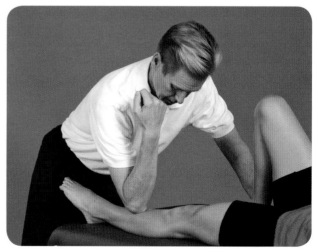

Figure 5.22

TIP It is obviously important to ensure that pain on the anterior shin is not the result of stress fractures, in which case this technique would be contraindicated.

Tight Calf Muscles

Many people suffer from tight calf muscles. The muscles in the posterior compartment of the leg bring about not only plantar flexion of the foot and ankle but also flexion of the knee (gastrocnemius), inversion of the foot and ankle (tibialis anterior and posterior), and flexion of the toes (the long toe flexors). It is not surprising that clients who engage in sporting activities that use the leg muscles may be prone to tension in these areas, as might people who wear high heels (which force the ankle into plantar flexion). Clients who remain seated for long periods of time may also experience shortening of tissues in this compartment because the gastrocnemius and the fascia associated with this part of the lower limb are held in a shortened position.

Active stretches

It could be argued that active stretches are more effective at combating tightness than passive stretches because the client is able to use body weight to facilitate the stretch. Good stretches include the standing calf stretches shown in figures 5.11 and 5.12. If a client finds these easy, suggest the stretches shown in figures 5.3 and 5.4, which place greater tension on tissues of the soleus.

Passive stretches

In addition to the stretches shown in figures 5.5, 5.6 and 5.14 for dorsiflexion of the ankle, soft tissue release to the calf is a good method for passively stretching this area. In this example (figure 5.23), the therapist is using the forearm to gently compress the tissues of the posterior calf. As he does this, he asks the client to dorsiflex the foot and ankle before moving on to a different position on the calf and once again compressing it gently.

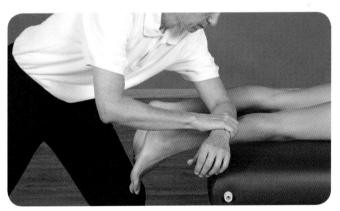

Figure 5.23

Cramp in the Calf

A cramp is an involuntary contraction, commonly felt in muscles of the calf, the exact cause of which is unknown. It is painful, aggravated by active or passive shortening of the muscle, and often experienced at night when the ankle naturally falls into a position of plantar flexion. Of short duration, it subsides naturally but is nevertheless painful and limits function.

Active stretches

Many people who suffer calf cramps know that by standing up and walking about, the cramp eventually subsides. During walking the foot is dorsiflexed, thus stretching the calf muscles. A useful way to combat a cramp is to contract the opposing muscle group, actively dorsiflexing the foot and ankle as in figure 5.7, inhibiting contraction in the muscles of the calf. The client should sustain this dorsiflexion until the cramp subsides. However, it can be challenging to dorsiflex the ankle through its entire range of motion, so using other stretches may be necessary. Examples of good stretches to help alleviate a cramp in the calf are shown in figures 5.3, 5.8, 5.10, 5.11 and 5.12.

Passive stretches

Passive stretches are useful if a cramp occurs during a massage treatment or if you happen to be treating a client before or after a sporting event. If the client is in the prone position, you could use the stretches shown in figures 5.5 and 5.6. If the client is in the supine position, use the stretch shown in figure 5.14.

Osteoarthritis in the Knee

Osteoarthritis is a wear-and-tear condition in which the hyaline cartilage of synovial joints degenerates as part of the natural aging process. It commonly occurs in older adults in the weight-bearing joints such as the hips, knees and lumbar spine. As the condition worsens, there is increasing pain, swelling and inflammation of the joint as more and more of the hyaline cartilage wears away. Degeneration of the hyaline cartilage covering the articulating bones of the knee joint is painful when the patient stands and during weight-bearing activities such as climbing or descending stairs, when the articulating surfaces of the knee joint grind together. Often such patients are advised to take part in exercises designed to strengthen the quadriceps and hamstrings, with the goal of providing extra muscular support to the joint. Such exercises might include non-weight-bearing activities such as cycling or swimming. Stretching the muscles of the quadriceps and hamstrings may soothe any tension that has built up in these muscles as a result of exercise.

Active stretches

Gentle stretching of the hamstrings and quadriceps is helpful for alleviating tension, although it is necessary to avoid pressure through the knee. Often the joint is swollen and painful to move. Whilst stretching is not a treatment per se for osteoarthritis of the knee, the movement required to perform some of the stretches helps increase synovial fluid in the joint and helps combat the muscular tension that may develop in patients enrolled in a lower limb strengthening programme before knee surgery for this particular condition. Ask your client to gently bend and straighten the leg while in the supine position, flexing and extending the knee as shown in figure 5.24. Flexion helps stretch the quadriceps, whilst extension tensions the popliteus, the hamstrings, the heads of the gastrocnemius and the fascia associated with these muscles.

Patients could also be encouraged to practise gentle knee flexion and extension stretches in water, provided these are deemed safe, because these too decrease weight bearing through the knee joint.

Passive stretches

You could start by assisting your client in knee flexion and extension in the supine position as shown in figure 5.24, gently adding pressure in the position of flexion providing this does not elicit pain. Alternatively, gentle tractioning of the lower limb helps stretch all lower limb tissues, including those of the knee joint, and may provide temporary relief. To do this, gently cup the client's ankle and apply slow, steady traction, one limb at a time, as shown in figure 5.25. Obviously, this also tractions the ankle and hip joints and cannot be performed if there are any acute conditions affecting either of these. Experiment in order to discover the handhold that works best for you.

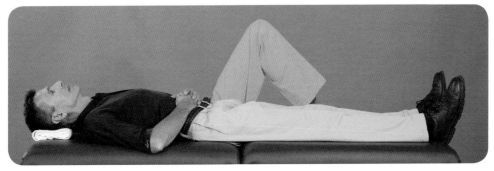

Figure 5.24

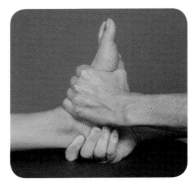

Figure 5.25

After Knee Surgery

Patients who have undergone surgery to the knee for conditions such as total or partial knee replacement, repair of cruciate ligaments or removal of a meniscus usually experience considerable swelling in the joint, which may have been immobilized after the operation. It is therefore not uncommon for such patients to experience stiffness in the knee and a decreased range of motion post-operatively. Both active and passive stretches are useful but should be carried out only once medical approval has been given.

Active stretches

Active flexion and extension movements within the patient's pain-free range will not only facilitate the lengthening of soft tissue structures in order to restore normal ROM at the knee but also help reduce swelling. The stretch shown in figure 5.24 is a good starting point. This could then be progressed to flexion and extension in a seated position. Or the patient could sit with the knee in extension, resting the calf and foot on a chair or stool in order to stretch the posterior capsule of the knee (figure 5.26). This is particularly helpful for

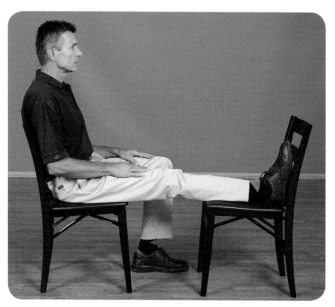

Figure 5.26

patients who have been unable to achieve full knee extension; in this position, gravity helps gently stretch the posterior of the joint.

Passive stretches

A simple passive stretch is to facilitate gentle flexion and extension of the knee (figure 5.27), supporting the lower limb beneath the knee and ankle as shown.

Passive knee flexion can also be encouraged in the prone position. However, some patients may feel uncomfortable in this position, particularly if they have an anterior scar that they feel anxious about resting on.

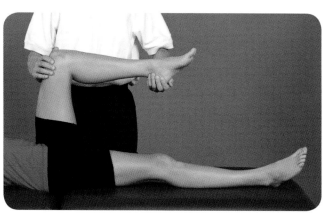

Figure 5.27

Hamstring Strain

Tears to hamstring muscles are common and frequently involve the proximal musculotendinous junction of the biceps femoris. Strains are classified as mild, moderate or severe. In mild strains, few muscle fibres are torn. Moderate strains cause damage to more fibres and a distinct loss of function; when severe, complete rupture of the muscle occurs. In addition to being very painful, moderate to severe strains are extremely disabling.

Acute

All forms of stretching are avoided during the early stages of tissue repair.

Sub-Acute

As with strains to other muscles, it is important to remember that pain subsides long before the healing process is complete. It is therefore wise to stretch conservatively during the sub-acute phase when there may be decreased pain and swelling.

Active stretches

Active stretches are particularly useful providing the client remains within a pain-free range. Begin with gentle stretches such as those shown in figures 5.7 and 5.10, which tension not only the tissues of the calf but also the hamstrings. Alternatively, use figure 5.26.

Passive stretches

Passive stretching is not recommended for hamstring strains.

Tight Hamstrings

There are many reasons for tightness to develop in the posterior thigh. It is commonly reported by runners and people regularly engaged in sports involving the lower limbs, such as tennis or rowing. Shortening of soft tissues of the posterior compartment of the thigh and knee is also likely to occur in people who remain seated for long periods of time, such as drivers, office workers or people who lead sedentary lifestyles. Both active and passive stretches are helpful in combating tight hamstrings.

Active stretches

There are a great many active hamstring stretches to choose from. These range from the simple sitting stretches shown in figures 5.7, 5.10 and 5.26 to standing stretches such as figure 5.11, which increases tension on the posterior thigh by also tensioning the calf muscles. In the supine position the client could use a towel, as in figure 5.28. Bear in mind that dorsiflexing the foot in this way also stretches the calf, and for some clients this may feel uncomfortable.

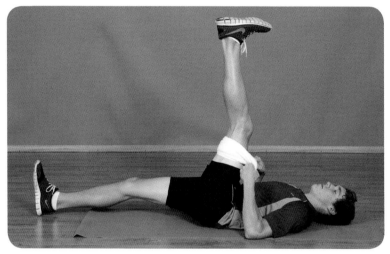

Figure 5.28

Remember that the hamstrings are hip extensors, so taking the hip into flexion, as in figure 5.29, will also help stretch these muscles. In this illustration the hamstrings of the *right* leg are being stretched because this is the hip that has been taken into flexion. Clients with knee problems should avoid this stretch, which places pressure on the knee opposite the thigh being stretched.

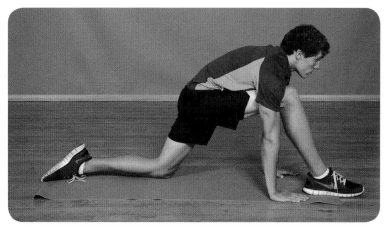

Figure 5.29

Clients who do not wish to do their stretches on the floor could simply try placing one leg on a stool and leaning forward to stretch the hamstrings of that limb. Obviously this is not appropriate for clients with impaired balance.

Less common but arguably just as effective ways to stretch the hamstrings are to apply active soft tissue release as in figures 5.30 and 5.31. Simply provide the client with a tennis ball, and show him how to position it against the thigh (as shown in figure 5.30) and then straighten the leg. The client can move the tennis ball to different positions on the hamstrings in this way, applying this technique for a few minutes each day.

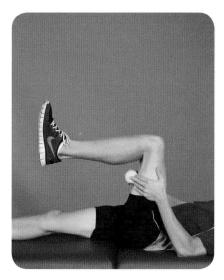

Figure 5.30

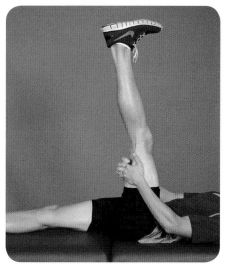

Figure 5.31

Passive stretches

Passive soft tissue release works well with the client in the prone position and is easy to apply. Simply start by shortening the hamstrings (figure 5.32) and choosing a place to gently compress these muscles. In this example the therapist has chosen to use his fist to apply the compression. Whilst maintaining this gentle compression, gently extend the knee, lowering the leg (figure 5.33). Repeat on another part of the muscle. You would not apply this stretching technique in the acute stage of injury or on clients you know bruise easily or are at risk of osteoporosis.

Alternatively, you could simply hold the client's leg in the position shown in figure 5.34, facilitating a stretch in the tissues of the posterior thigh. You could use this as the starting position to perform muscle energy technique (MET), following the protocol described in chapter 4 (page 44). The leg that is not being stretched could be extended as shown here, or the knee can be allowed to remain flexed if extension is uncomfortable, taking pressure off the lumbar spine.

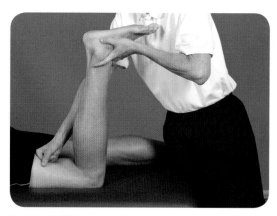

Figure 5.32

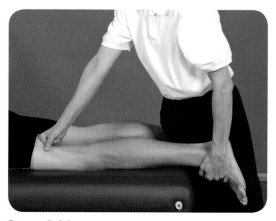

Figure 5.33

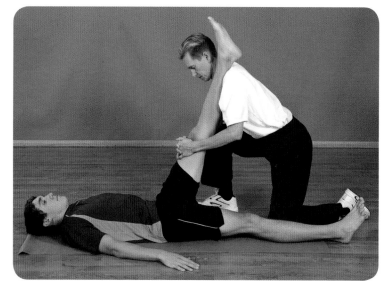

Figure 5.34

Hamstring Cramp

Involuntary contraction in the hamstrings is painful albeit temporary. Cramping is more likely to occur after vigorous physical exertion or in patients who remain positioned for long periods of time in knee flexion. Although both active and passive stretches are helpful, active stretches may be the most beneficial because contraction of the quadriceps or hip flexors inhibits the hamstrings, which therefore cannot contract involuntarily (i.e., cramp).

Active stretches

Stretches in figures 5.3, 5.7, 5.10, 5.11 and 5.12 are all helpful in combating hamstring cramps.

Passive stretches

Sometimes hamstrings cramp when clients are lying prone and actively flex their knees, or more commonly when receiving massage in this position after a sporting event. In either case it is useful to have some stretches to help overcome this.

If the cramp occurs when the client is prone, flex the knee and ask her to push her ankle into your hand (figure 5.35), contracting her quadriceps. Contraction of the quadriceps in this way inhibits the hamstrings and helps reduce the cramp. Ask her to push her leg back down onto the therapy couch (or floor if you are working on the floor) as you apply gentle resistance.

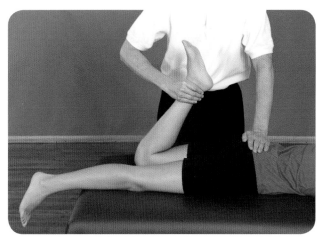

Figure 5.35

If hamstrings cramp when the client is seated, apply the same technique. Place your hand over the ankle of the leg that is cramping, and ask the client to try to straighten her leg, pushing against you (figure 5.36) until the knee is extended. As with the previous stretch, contraction of the quadriceps in this way inhibits contraction of the hamstrings.

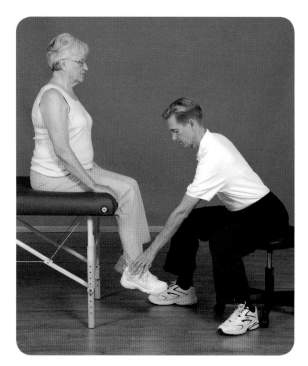

Figure 5.36

Groin Strain

Groin strains are particularly common in sports where muscles such as adductor longus or gracilis may be damaged by impact, sudden contraction or overstretching.

Acute

All forms of stretching should be avoided during the early stages of tissue repair.

Sub-Acute

Stretching should be conservative in order to prevent reinjury to muscles not yet fully healed.

Active stretches

Groin strains can take a long time to heal; therefore, implementation of an early active stretching programme is recommended providing this does not cause pain. Lying on a bed or on the floor, a client could begin by gently abducting the legs (with the knees extended). If this is tolerable, she could progress to sitting cross-legged (figure 5.37). If this is uncomfortable, the client could place pillows beneath each knee for support. Once this is tolerable, she could progress to figure 5.38. To increase the stretch in either 5.37 or 5.38, the client simply places gentle downward pressure on the knees.

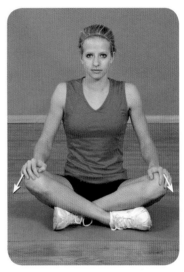

Figure 5.37

An alternative adductor stretch is figure 5.39. To increase this stretch the client simply leans forwards; to decrease it she leans backwards. Note that this stretch also requires flexibility in the hamstrings.

Passive stretches

Passive stretches are not recommended for groin strains.

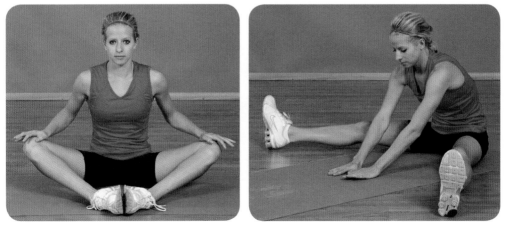

Figure 5.38

Figure 5.39

Tight Adductors

People who engage in sporting activities such as running, football and swimming often think it is beneficial to stretch their adductor muscles as part of their cool-down programme of stretches, or simply to decrease sensations of stiffness after exercise. Adductors contract as we walk, and so people who walk a lot as part of their general lifestyle or fitness activities may also benefit from stretching these muscles. Adductors may become tight after periods of immobility, leading to muscle imbalance in the pelvis and lower limbs.

Active stretches

Each of the stretches shown in figures 5.37, 5.38 and 5.39 are helpful for combating tight adductors. Others include those shown in figures 5.40 and 5.41. Obviously the stretch shown in figure 5.40 is not suitable for clients with balance problems, and the stretch shown in figure 5.41 places pressure on the knee of the leg not being stretched, so it is not suitable for all clients. Both of these stretches are safe, but bear in mind that they place more pressure on the medial collateral ligaments of the knee than the stretches shown in figures 5.37 and 5.38.

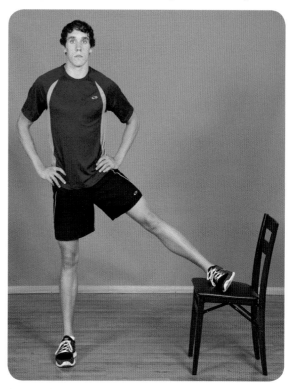

Figure 5.40

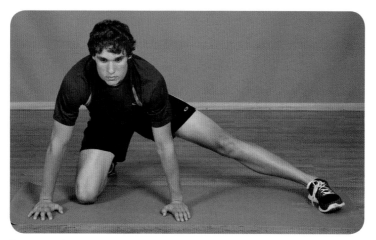

Figure 5.41

Passive stretches

Useful passive adductor stretches are shown in figures 5.42 and figure 5.43. Notice how in figure 5.42 the therapist prevents the pelvis from moving by gently placing pressure on the anterior superior iliac spine. This can be uncomfortable for some clients, so you might want to place a sponge or small towel between your hand and the client's hip. In figure 5.43 the therapist is abducting the leg whilst being sure to support the knee. Notice that in this position, extension of the lumbar spine may be exaggerated, and this is a position that may aggravate back pain in some subjects.

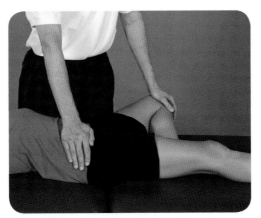

Figure 5.42

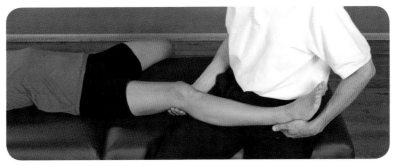

Figure 5.43

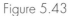 Notice how in figure 5.43 the leg that is not being stretched has been hooked over one side of the treatment couch. This prevents the client from being pulled to one side of the couch. First check that this position is comfortable, and perhaps insert a sponge between the client's knee and the side of the couch.

Tight Quadriceps

The quadriceps may be tight as a result of a sporting activity or after injury. Both active and passive stretches are helpful.

Active stretches

The quadriceps can be actively stretched in the lying (figure 5.44) or standing (figure 5.45) position. In each, the client needs to be able to reach behind herself to hold her ankle, and this requires good flexibility in the muscles of the chest and anterior shoulder joint. The standing stretch is not appropriate for clients with poor balance or who cannot bear weight through their hip, knee or ankle. To make this stretch safer, ask the client to perform it whilst supporting herself against a wall or placing one hand on a table for balance. The stretch in figure 5.44 could also be performed in the side-lying position.

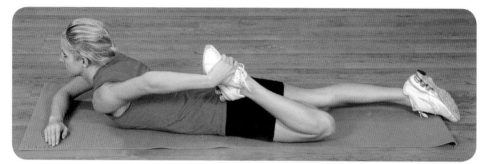

Figure 5.44

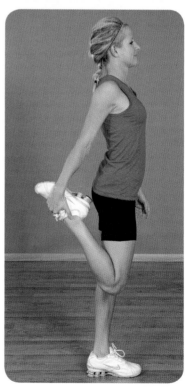

TIP Pressing the pelvis forward (flattening the lumbar spine in a posterior pelvic tilt) increases the stretch in both positions.

Figure 5.45

Passive stretches

The stretch shown in figure 5.46 is a common way to passively stretch the quadriceps. The quadriceps may also be stretched in the supine position (figure 5.47), provided clients are comfortable in this position. If a client has very tight quadriceps, they may be stretched with the client in a seated position. Simply kneel down, and placing your hand on the client's ankle, gently flex the knee.

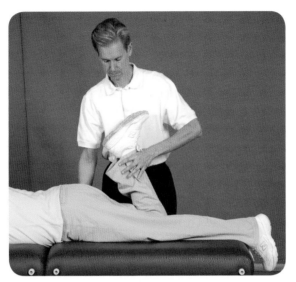

Figure 5.46

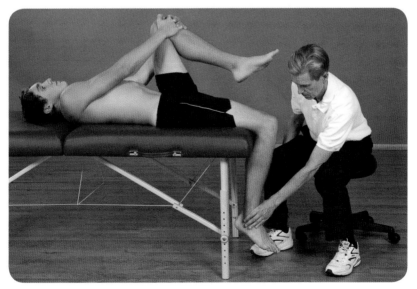

Figure 5.47

 TIP To enhance the stretch in figure 5.46, stabilize the pelvis by placing a bolster or folded towel over the sacrum and resting on it as you flex the knee.

Tight Hip Flexors

The hip flexors include the psoas, iliacus and rectus femoris, all of which may feel tight after prolonged hip flexion or sporting activity.

Active stretches

Figure 5.48 illustrates how to stretch the hip flexor by hanging the affected leg off one side of a bed. Kneeling (figure 5.49) is an alternative for those clients who are comfortable on their knees like this. In both positions, flattening the low back so the pelvis is posteriorly tilted increases the stretch on the hip flexors. An easy way to explain this is to suggest that the client contract the buttock muscles.

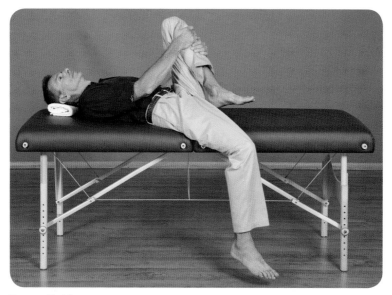

Figure 5.48

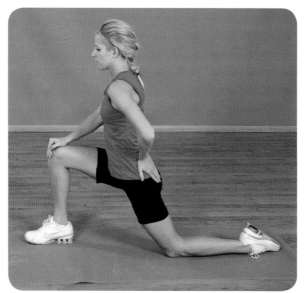

Figure 5.49

TIP The stretch shown in figure 5.49 can be further enhanced by the client's raising his arm above his head and turning towards the flexed knee of the opposite leg (figure 5.50). In this way all the fascia connecting the anterior hip and thigh and the lateral side of the body is tensioned.

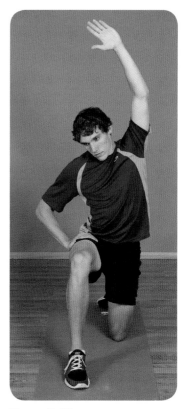

Figure 5.50

Passive stretches

Passive stretches for the hip flexors could be performed in the prone (figure 5.51) or supine (figure 5.52) position. To perform the stretch with the client prone, a small towel needs to be inserted beneath the knee in order to take the hip into slight extension. In some clients, this increases lordosis in the lumbar spine and may be uncomfortable. Stabilize the pelvis to prevent movement during the stretch. Notice that in stretch 5.52 the client needs to be positioned in such a way as to be able to extend the hip (thereby stretching the flexors of the hip) and not have the thigh supported as in this photo.

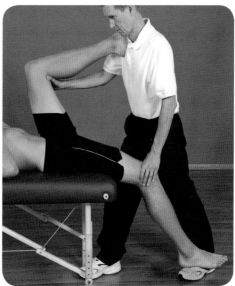

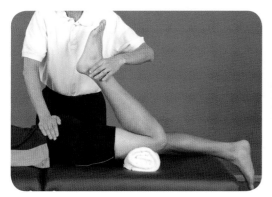

Figure 5.51

Figure 5.52

Iliotibial Band Friction Syndrome (Runner's Knee)

It is not entirely clear what causes the lateral knee pain experienced by some runners and popularly referred to as *runner's knee*. Some believe the pain is due to tissues of the lateral thigh rubbing against the epicondyle of the femur and have postulated that stretching these will alleviate pain.

Active stretches

Many people advocate stretching the iliotibial band (ITB) using foam rollers (figure 5.53). Because the gluteus maximus inserts into the ITB, it may be that stretching this muscle (see figures 5.55 and 5.56) will also help reduce tension in the lateral thigh.

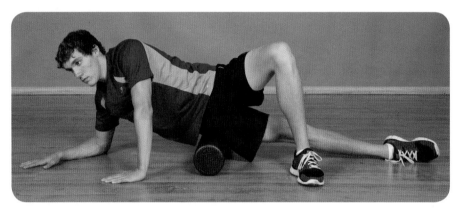

Figure 5.53

Passive stretches

If you think that passive stretching of the ITB is workable, try the stretch shown in figure 5.54 with the client in the side-lying position. Be careful when performing this stretch as it requires the client to be positioned close to the edge of the treatment couch. As with active stretches, stretching muscles of the buttock (see figure 5.57), which include the piriformis, may decrease tension in tissues of the lateral thigh.

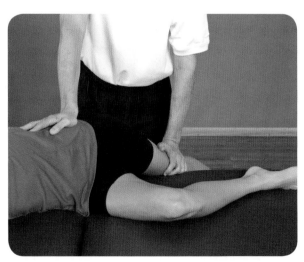

Figure 5.54

Piriformis Syndrome

This is the name given to pain in the buttocks and lower limb resulting from compression of the sciatic nerve by the piriformis muscle.

Active stretches

Two useful active stretches for the gluteal area are shown in figures 5.55 and 5.56. These also tension the iliotibial band and may be useful in alleviating muscular tension in the lateral thigh.

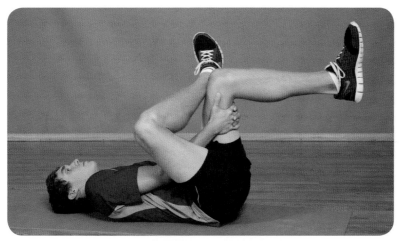

Figure 5.55

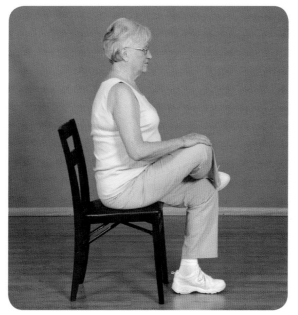

Figure 5.56

Passive stretches

The passive stretch shown in figure 5.57 is useful but difficult to apply with a client on a treatment couch because of the force needed to stretch the strong muscles of the buttock region. Start with the hip and knee of the client at 90-degree angles as shown here, and move the lower limb towards the client in an attempt to bring about a stretch in the gluteal region. Solicit feedback from your client to help determine the best position to hold the stretch. Some clients find this position uncomfortable when it compresses the rectus femoris tendon on the anterior of the hip.

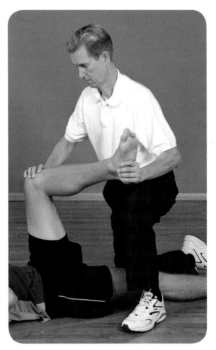

Figure 5.57

Delayed Onset Muscle Soreness

DOMS is a sensation of soreness often experienced after a period of intense physical activity or physical activity the client is not used to performing. It is characterized by mild soreness and some stiffening of soft tissues the day after exertion, with the muscles becoming intensely sore and painful to both touch and movement (both active and passive) 48 hours later. The condition subsides naturally. The exact mechanisms of DOMS are unknown, although it is believed to involve microtrauma to the involved muscle tissue. This is a short-lived condition, the characteristics of which some people believe are moderated by stretching, either actively or passively. Stretching recommendations are to treat as for a sub-acute muscle strain because forceful stretching could have a negative effect on muscles suffering microtrauma. Therefore if you are treating someone with DOMS in the lower limbs, refer to stretches for sub-acute strains to the calf, hamstrings, quadriceps or adductors, selecting whichever seem most appropriate.

Quick Questions

1. Look at table 5.1. Which stretches are the safest for treating sub-acute injuries, active or passive?
2. Why is it useful to use calf stretches (both active and passive) when treating clients with plantar fasciitis?
3. Why are active stretches good to recommend to clients suffering calf or hamstring cramps?
4. When performing passive adductor stretches in the supine position, what do you need to do to the client's pelvis?
5. How do you prevent the pelvis from tilting when performing passive stretches to the quadriceps in the prone position?

Stretching the Upper Limb

The material within this chapter will help you identify stretches to use when rehabilitating clients with conditions affecting the upper limbs. Table 6.1 lists the conditions included within this chapter and which stretches might be helpful. Altogether, the chapter discusses 42 stretches, 23 active and 19 passive. In table 6.1, you will find stretches that may help with the rehabilitation of clients with injuries, such as a sprained wrist or rotator cuff strain, as well as more long-term conditions, such as a stiff shoulder. Information is also provided on stretching after mastectomy, which will help you appreciate how stretching is used post-surgically.

Note: The stretches listed in this table for each pathology are not the *only* stretches that could or should be used. Within each section you will often find tips for modifying a stretch or recommendations to include stretches shown in other parts of this chapter. Additional useful stretches for each pathology are shown in *italics* within table 6.1. The numbers in the table (e.g., 6.1, 6.2) refer to the figure numbers that illustrate the stretch.

Table 6.1   Stretches for the Upper Limb

	Active	Passive
SHOULDER		
Adhesive capsulitis (frozen shoulder)	6.1, page 89 6.2, page 90 6.3, page 90 6.4, page 90	6.5, page 91 6.6, page 91 6.7, page 91
Stiff shoulder	6.8, page 92 6.9, page 92 *6.1, page 89* *6.2, page 90* *6.3, page 90* *6.4, page 90*	6.10, page 93 6.11, page 93 6.12, page 93 6.13, page 94 *6.5, page 91* *6.6, page 91* *6.7, page 91* *6.16, page 96*

»*continued*

»continued

	Active	Passive
SHOULDER		
Shortened internal rotators of the humerus	6.14, page 95 6.15, page 95	6.16, page 96 *6.10, page 93* *6.13, page 94*
Rotator cuff strain: acute	Not recommended	Not recommended
Rotator cuff strain: sub-acute	6.17, page 97 *Providing these are pain-free positions:* *6.1, page 89* *6.2, page 90* *6.3, page 90* *6.4, page 90*	6.18, page 98
Supraspinatus tendinosis: acute	Not recommended	Not recommended
Supraspinatus tendinosis: sub-acute	6.19, page 99	6.20, page 100 *6.10, page 93*
After mastectomy	6.21, page 101 6.22, page 101 *6.1, page 89* *6.2, page 90* *6.3, page 90* *6.4, page 90*	*6.5, page 91* *6.6, page 91* *6.7, page 91*
ELBOW		
Lateral epicondylitis (tennis elbow)	6.23, page 102	6.24, page 102
Medial epicondylitis (golfer's elbow)	6.25, page 103 6.26, page 103	6.27, page 103
Stiff elbow	6.28, page 104 6.29, page 104	6.30, page 105 6.31, page 105
WRIST, HAND AND FINGERS		
Sprained wrist: acute	Not recommended	Not recommended
Sprained wrist: sub-acute	6.32, page 106 6.33, page 106 *6.34, page 107* *6.35, page 107* *6.36, page 107*	Not recommended
Stiff wrist and fingers	6.34, page 107 6.35, page 107 6.36, page 107 *6.32, page 106* *6.33, page 106*	6.37, page 108 6.38, page 108 6.39, page 108 6.40, page 108
Carpal tunnel syndrome	6.41, page 109	6.42, page 109 *6.37, page 108*

Adhesive Capsulitis (Frozen Shoulder)

This painful condition has no known cause and is characterized by the gradual onset of stiffness and pain in the shoulder. Range of motion in the glenohumeral joint becomes increasingly restricted, especially abduction and lateral rotation. Similar to Dupuytren's contracture in the hand, in late stages of adhesive capsulitis it appears that the restriction in movement is largely due to the secretion of excessive amounts of collagen. This in turn leads to contractures in soft tissues such as the coracohumeral ligament and subscapularis muscle. It is not clear whether active or passive stretching is better, although both may be of help.

Active stretches

Swinging the arm in a pendulum-like motion as in figure 6.1 may help maintain range of motion by gently tractioning the soft tissues of the shoulder joint. A light weight could be added if necessary. It is useful to have a table on which a client may rest to prevent straining the low back in this position.

TIP Observe the degree of shoulder flexion required to perform this pendulum movement. In this illustration it is almost 90 degrees. Not all clients can tolerate this degree of flexion and will need to start in a more upright position, the arm held closer to the body. As a client is able to tolerate increasing flexion at the waist, so, too, does the degree of shoulder flexion increase.

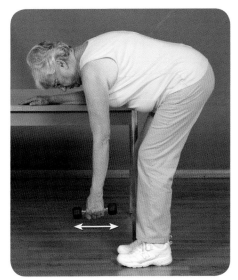

Figure 6.1

An interesting and safe way to help clients improve flexion at the shoulder (by stretching the adductor muscles and tissues of the armpit) is to show them how to slide a plastic bag across a tabletop (figure 6.2). In this manner, they are not required to hold up their arms against gravity.

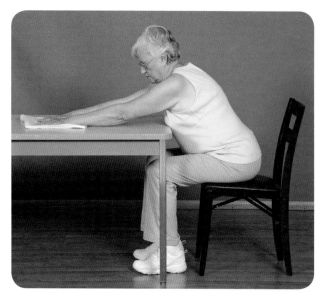

Figure 6.2

Another way to maintain and improve abduction is to suggest that when resting, a client sit with a small cushion under the arm as in figure 6.3. This helps gently stretch the soft tissues of the armpit, including the adductor muscles. As abduction increases, the stretch could be modified so the client has a larger cushion or rests the arm on a table as in figure 6.4.

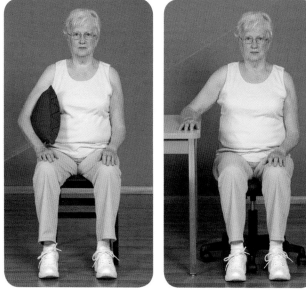

Figure 6.3   Figure 6.4

Passive stretches

With all these stretches it is important to remember that adhesive capsulitis can be extremely painful. It is therefore prudent to provide one stretch of limited duration and to check with the patient the following day about what effect this had.

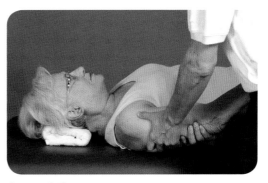

Figure 6.5

A simple starting point is to gently traction the soft tissues of the glenohumeral joint, supporting the arm as shown in figure 6.5. Remember that range of motion is restricted, so abduction may be difficult or painful. It is often necessary to keep the arm supported, close to the body. Notice too how the therapist in this illustration is holding the arm in such a way as to localize the stretch to the shoulder joint. Experiment to determine the handhold that works best for you and the client.

This stretch may also be performed with the client seated (figure 6.6). The disadvantage is that the client may not relax as much as when the same stretch is performed in the supine position. When seated, there is also a tendency for the client to lean towards the side being stretched, whereas when supine, the arm may be tractioned against the weight of the body.

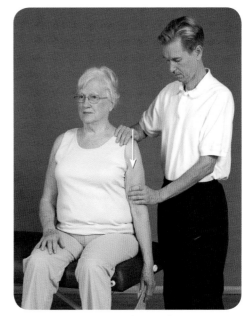

Figure 6.6

In later stages of the condition, when ROM is improving, it is likely that manual therapists may perform a range of accessory movements to facilitate the rehabilitation of a patient recovering from frozen shoulder. One such movement that might be safely incorporated as an initial stretch is to apply gentle pressure to the anterior surface of the shoulder (figure 6.7). This stretches the soft tissues of the anterior joint and may help increase range in the joint if the stretch brings about an accessory glide (i.e., a movement of the head of the humerus from the anterior to posterior position against the glenohumeral joint).

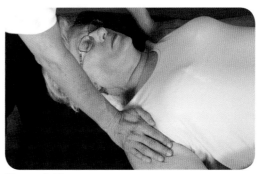

Figure 6.7

Stiff Shoulder

All the stretches in the previous section on adhesive capsulitis may be helpful if a client has a very stiff shoulder. Other useful stretches are shown here. These assume the client has a greater degree of abduction and lateral rotation than might be expected in a patient with adhesive capsulitis.

Active stretches

In addition to the stretches in the section for adhesive capsulitis (figures 6.1, 6.2, 6.3 and 6.4), the client could try those shown in figures 6.8 and 6.9. In figure 6.8 a towel is used, the subject using the left arm to help improve range of motion in the right shoulder by gently drawing the right hand up the back. In figure 6.9 the client simply uses body weight against a broom handle to stretch the inferior capsule of the joint, an area that often becomes tight when a person has been using crutches, isometrically contracting the adductor muscles.

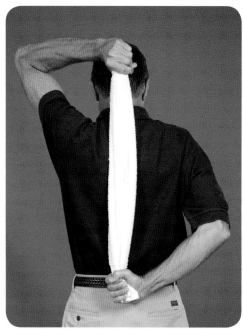

Figure 6.8

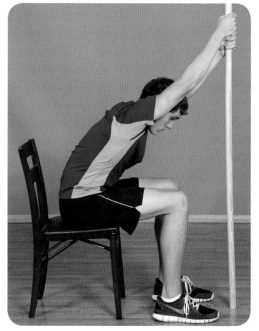

Figure 6.9

Passive stretches

Stretches shown in figures 6.5, 6.6 and 6.7 are all good starting stretches. A variant of the stretch shown in figure 6.5 is to apply gentle traction to the shoulder and then ask the client to slowly turn her head away from you (laterally flexing the neck), taking her ear to her shoulder as in figure 6.10. Because muscles and fascia connect the head, neck and shoulder, moving the head in this way tensions the soft tissues of the shoulder to a greater extent than if you were to apply *only* traction or if the client were to *only* flex the neck.

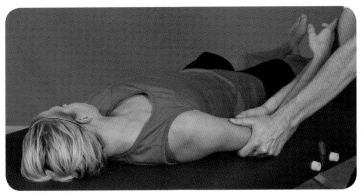

Figure 6.10

TIP It is important that as the therapist, you apply gentle traction first, before the client moves her head. In this way it is the client who is in charge of the stretch.

Another way to improve range in this joint is to apply traction in a variety of positions. For example, try 90 degrees of flexion with the client supine (figure 6.11) or prone (figure 6.12). (Also consider using figure 6.16 if the tissues restrict external rotation of this joint.) With all of these stretches, practice using different handholds to avoid tractioning the elbow joint.

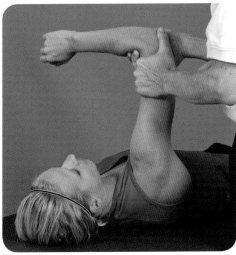

Figure 6.11

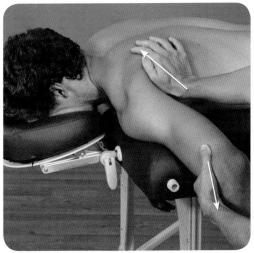

Figure 6.12

Take care stretching the internal rotators of the humerus (figure 6.13). Only gentle overpressure is needed against the wrist to encourage the tissues restricting external rotation to lengthen.

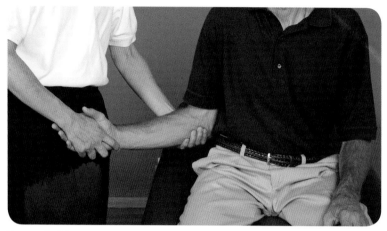

Figure 6.13

 Sometimes, alternating between stretches 6.13 and 6.6 can help increase range in a stiff shoulder joint.

Shortened Internal Rotators of the Humerus

Clients with kyphotic postures or those engaged in sports that involve throwing often have shortness in the internal rotators of the humerus. Internal rotators include teres major and subscapularis, as well as the anterior fibres of the deltoid plus pectoralis major.

Active stretches

Exercises that help strengthen the external rotators will also help decrease tone in the internal rotators and can be a good adjunct to a stretching programme. Examples of such exercises are shown in figures 6.14 and 6.15. Pulling on a resistance band to activate muscles such as infraspinatus may help inhibit the internal rotators and would therefore be helpful before applying passive stretch 6.13, for example.

TIP Note that the movements shown in figures 6.14 and 6.15 are different; in figure 6.14 the arm is adducted, whereas in figure 6.15 it is abducted. Some clients will feel more comfortable with the arm adducted, others with it abducted.

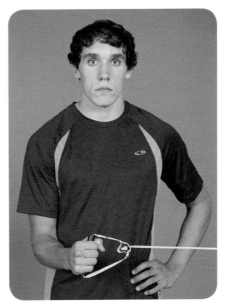

Figure 6.14

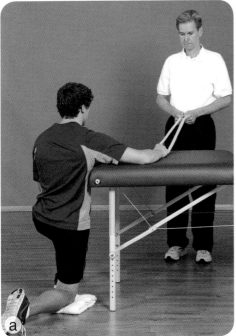 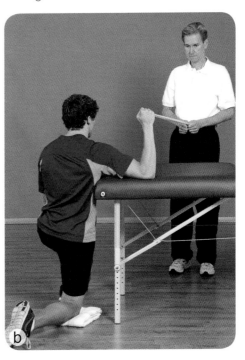

Figure 6.15

Passive stretches

One way to combat shortened internal rotators is to apply stretches that both traction the shoulder (figure 6.10) and stretch the rotators themselves (figure 6.16). In this example the arm is abducted to 90 degrees, but not all clients will feel comfortable with this degree of abduction if the shoulder is stiff.

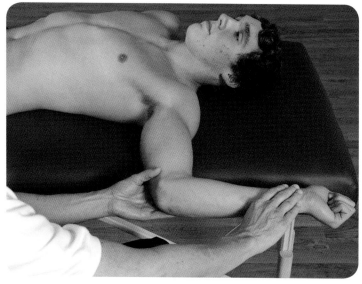

Figure 6.16

 TIP This is a good starting position for the application of muscle energy technique (MET). Refer to the protocol on page 44 to see how MET might work in this position to help stretch the internal rotators of the humerus.

Rotator Cuff Strain

Muscles of the rotator cuff are supraspinatus, infraspinatus, teres minor and subscapularis. Tears in one or more of these muscles are common in the sporting population, especially in athletes using repetitive overhead motion of the arm. Elderly people sometimes complain of severe shoulder pain with no history of trauma or overuse and on examination are found to have rotator cuff tears. It is not clear why older adults sustain these tears, but the cause could be reduced blood flow associated with the normal degenerative process. It is important to remember that in addition to restoring normal range of motion, during rehabilitation subjects are likely to be engaged in activities designed to help restore strength and control of their muscles and overall stabilization of the shoulder joint.

Acute

The acute stage is deemed to be when there is inflammation or pain. Stretching is not recommended at this stage.

Sub-Acute

When there is a reduction in pain and inflammation, gentle stretching, applied cautiously, may be helpful in maintaining and regaining ROM.

Active stretches

All the active stretches in the section on adhesive capsulitis may be helpful in the sub-acute stages of rotator cuff strain (see figures 6.1, 6.2, 6.3 and 6.4). Pendulum movements or any form of self-tractioning should be gentle and minimal. In addition, it is important to stretch the posterior capsule of the shoulder as in figure 6.17 providing there is no pain.

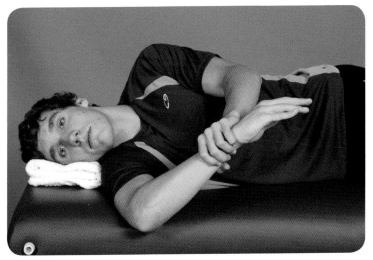

Figure 6.17

Passive stretches

With the client positioned as shown in figure 6.18, gently take the arm into internal rotation to stretch the posterior capsule. Remember that this stretch is to be performed only in later stages of rehabilitation and providing there is no pain.

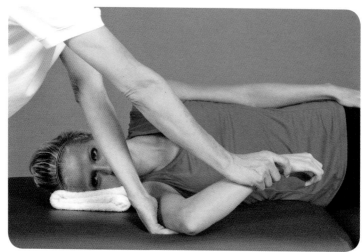

Figure 6.18

Supraspinatus Tendinosis

Damage to the supraspinatus tendon is common in athletes who engage in sports that use repetitive overhead arm movements, such as baseball, tennis and swimming. It is a difficult muscle to stretch in isolation because it is both a stabilizer of the humeral head and an abductor of the arm as well as part of the rotator cuff. Stretching the supraspinatus necessitates traction plus adduction, a challenging position to attain.

Acute

Stretching the supraspinatus is not recommended if there is pain or inflammation.

Sub-Acute

It may be useful to begin a stretching programme in the sub-acute stage when there is a reduction in pain.

Active stretches

Adducting the arm with or without lateral neck flexion (figure 6.19) might be helpful. In this photo the subject is attempting to stretch the supraspinatus muscle of the right shoulder and is performing lateral neck flexion to the left to further enhance the stretch in soft tissues.

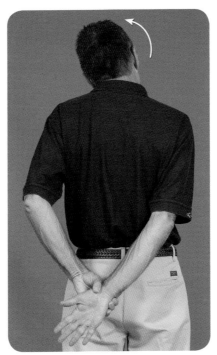

Figure 6.19

Passive stretches

Because the supraspinatus is wrapped in fascia that is consistent with fascia of the neck, a starting point might be to try gentle shoulder traction with lateral neck flexion as in figure 6.10. Another approach is to locate the muscle beneath the upper fibres of the trapezius (figure 6.20). Then apply static pressure to part of it. As you do so, ask the client to depress the shoulder, drawing the hand towards the feet. Your pressure acts as a kind of soft tissue release, locking part of the soft tissues to underlying structures.

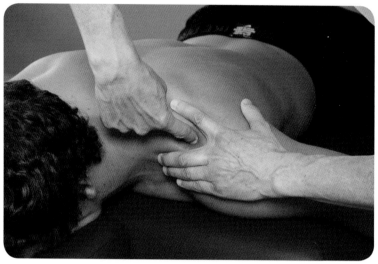

Figure 6.20

After Mastectomy

There are various types of mastectomy and various surgical approaches, so as with any post-surgical therapy, it is important to follow the guidance of the surgeon in charge and to follow the therapeutic protocol of the hospital or clinic where the operation was performed and where the client is recovering. Anxiety after the operation may leave some women fearful of abducting their arm. It may be held or strapped protectively against the body in the early stages of recovery. However, maintenance of this posture may lead to shortening and tightening of fascia and soft tissues of the shoulder, chest and neck, and this can be detrimental to proper functioning later on. It is therefore important to gain the confidence of the client and to encourage her to follow the stretching protocol that may be in place. Such a protocol may include the kinds of stretches shown here.

Active stretches

The active stretches in the section on adhesive capsulitis are helpful in the early stages of post-mastectomy rehabilitation for regaining range of motion in the shoulder joint (see figures 6.1, 6.2, 6.3 and 6.4). In addition, walking the arm up the wall as in figures 6.21 and 6.22 will help improve flexion and abduction, respectively.

Passive stretches

Providing you have medical approval for stretching, stretches such as those shown in figures 6.5, 6.6 and 6.7 might be beneficial when working with women after mastectomy.

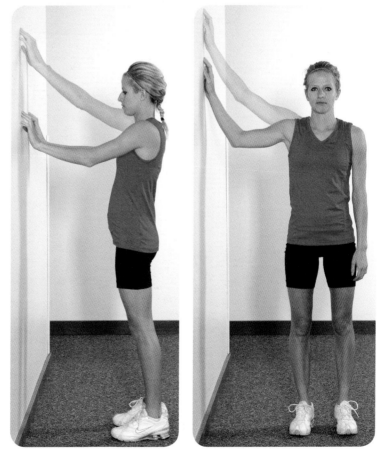

Figure 6.21   Figure 6.22

Lateral Epicondylitis (Tennis Elbow)

Lateral epicondylitis, popularly known as tennis elbow, is a painful condition resulting from overuse of the extensor muscles of the wrist, characterized by pain over the common extensor origin of the lateral epicondyle of the humerus. Rest is commonly advocated, with restricted use of the wrist and avoidance of elbow extension. Stretching may help maintain wrist and elbow range of motion but more important may help reduce pain.

Active stretches

Demonstrate to your client how to stretch the wrist extensors as shown in figure 6.23, keeping the elbow extended. Performing the stretch with the elbow flexed is not as powerful because the wrist extensor muscles originate on the lateral epicondyle, superior to the elbow joint. However, if the stretch is painful with the elbow in extension, begin with the elbow flexed.

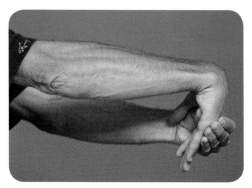

Figure 6.23

Passive stretches

Passive stretches can be done in either the seated (figure 6.24) or supine position.

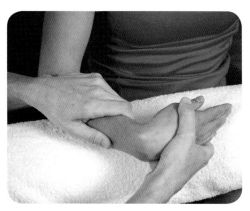

Figure 6.24

TIP If you wish to perform the stretch with the client prone, simply ensure his wrist is able to flex by positioning him with his arms abducted and over his head, his hands resting over the edge of the couch.

Medial Epicondylitis (Golfer's Elbow)

Overuse of the flexor muscles of the wrist and fingers may lead to medial epicondylitis, more commonly known as golfer's elbow and characterized by pain at the common flexor origin at the medial epicondyle.

Active stretches

Examples of useful active stretches for medial epicondylitis are shown in figures 6.25 and 6.26. These stretches are easily modified so that a client rests her palm against a wall or even a table. Stretching with the palms against a table enables the subject to bear weight through the elbow and wrist joints, something that may be desirable towards the end of the rehabilitative process.

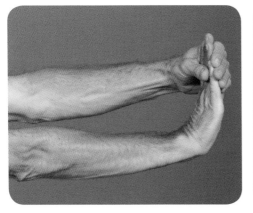

Figure 6.25

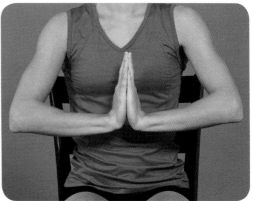

Figure 6.26

Passive stretches

Similar to passive stretching of the extensor muscles for lateral epicondylitis, stretching the wrist flexor muscles can be performed with the client seated (as shown in figure 6.27) or supine. Fully extending the elbow and fingers increases the stretch.

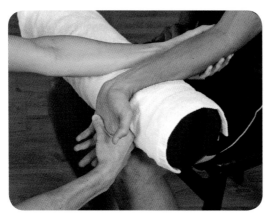

Figure 6.27

Stiff Elbow

Stiffness in this joint is common not only after surgery to the area but also after immobilization of the upper limb for conditions such as fracture to the humerus. In attempting to increase movement at the elbow, it is important to include the movements of supination and pronation, not just those of flexion and extension.

Active stretches

Patients may facilitate improvements in range of motion by performing extension and flexion of the elbow, trying to ensure they fully extend or fully flex the joint. One way to make this movement easier is for the patient to rest the arm on a table whilst performing the stretch, as in figure 6.28, or to use the other hand to facilitate the stretch, as in figure 6.29.

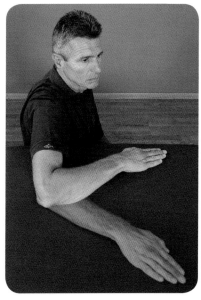

Figure 6.28   Figure 6.29

Passive stretches

Passive flexion and extension of the elbow joint (figure 6.30) is easy to perform and will help maintain or increase range of motion at this joint. Passive supination and pronation may be added as you take the elbow through its normal range. One way to do this is to hold the patient's hand as shown in figure 6.31.

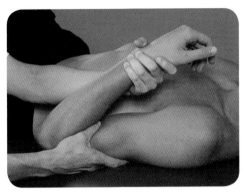

Figure 6.30

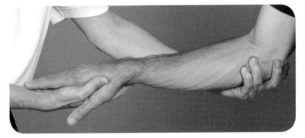

Figure 6.31

Sprained Wrist

Sprain to the ligaments of the wrist is a common injury affecting athletes and non-athletes alike. It commonly occurs during sport where a subject falls onto an outstretched hand, or in the elderly slipping in poor weather. Immobilization to allow healing is common, either in bandages or a splint, with the arm held protectively in a sling. In severe cases involving fracture, the wrist may be cast. As a consequence of immobilization, the soft tissues of the wrist may stiffen, restricting flexion, extension, radial deviation and ulnar deviation. There may also be restriction in supination and pronation. It is important to compare the left and right wrists for ROM as this is quite variable and may be decreased in older adults.

Acute

Stretching is not recommended for acute wrist sprains.

Sub-Acute

Gentle stretching may be helpful if started during the sub-acute stage when pain and swelling have subsided. Take care when advising clients because ligaments take weeks to heal, and stretching should be conservative in order to prevent reinjury.

Active stretches

Active stretching is necessary to help regain ROM. There are four movements to maintain: flexion and extension (figure 6.32) and radial and ulnar deviation (figure 6.33). Note that these ranges are likely to be severely decreased after wrist sprain, due to an increase in tissue swelling and contracture of soft tissues. Simple active stretches involve the client practising these four movements. Flexing the wrist stretches the wrist and finger extensor muscles; extending the wrist stretches the flexors of the wrist and fingers. Deviation of the wrist to the radial side of the forearm stretches the muscles of ulnar deviation; deviation of the wrist to the ulnar side of the forearm stretches the muscles of radial deviation. Clients should start with movements of small amplitude, within their pain-free range, gradually increasing their range of motion over time. Active flexion and extension movements are performed first as these are likely to be easier to perform than ulnar and radial deviation.

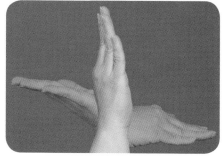

Figure 6.32

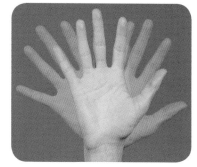

Figure 6.33

TIP   It is also important to stretch the fingers (see figures 6.34, 6.35 and 6.36) because the long tendons of the finger flexors and finger extensors cross the wrist joint.

Passive stretches

Passive stretching is not recommended for sub-acute wrist sprains.

Stiff Wrist and Fingers

Like other joints, a wrist may stiffen after injury or immobility. Both active and passive stretches are helpful in increasing ROM and stretching the associated muscles.

Active stretches

Start with the stretches shown in figures 6.32 and 6.33 to improve wrist ROM. To improve extension of both the wrist and fingers, progress to interlinking the fingers as in figure 6.34.

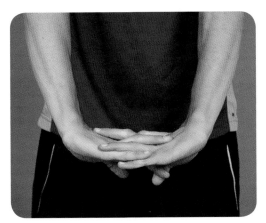

Figure 6.34

Aids are helpful here too. For example, using a tennis ball is helpful at stretching the flexor tendons of the fingers and wrist (figure 6.35). By comparison, using a band as in figure 6.36 can help improve flexion of the fingers, stretching the extensor tendons.

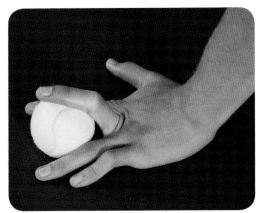

Figure 6.35

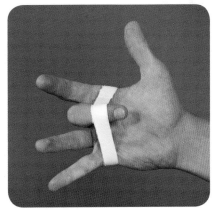

Figure 6.36

Passive stretches

Passive traction of the wrist (figure 6.37) could be performed, as could flexion (figure 6.38), extension (figure 6.39), and radial and ulnar deviation (figure 6.40). Passively extending the fingers as in figure 6.39 increases the stretch on the wrist flexor tendons and can be included once wrist extension has been regained.

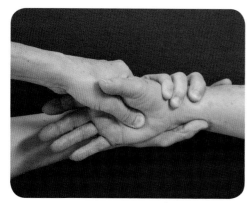

Figure 6.37

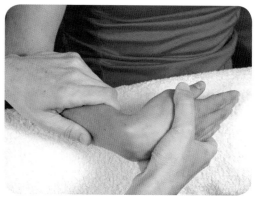

Figure 6.38

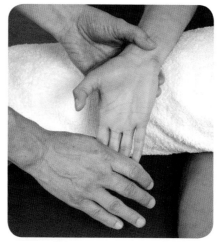

Figure 6.39

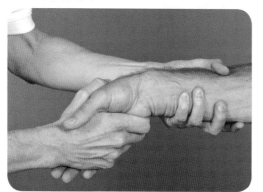

Figure 6.40

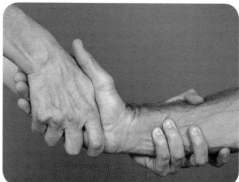

Carpal Tunnel Syndrome

Carpal tunnel syndrome is the name of a condition involving impairment of the median nerve as it passes through the carpal tunnel, formed by the eight small bones that make up the wrist. The condition is believed to be caused by a build-up of pressure within the carpal tunnel, leading to ischemia of the nerve. This in turn leads to pain and impairment of the hand and fingers, often with accompanying pain in the forearm. Stretching the soft tissues of the forearm, wrist and fingers may help alleviate pressure within the carpal tunnel and may therefore be a useful adjunct to more invasive treatments. However, subjects often experience numbness, tingling and pain with this condition, so any passive stretching needs to be cautious, with the therapist soliciting feedback from the client throughout. It is important not to exacerbate symptoms. Because each case is different, it seems prudent to try a small amount of stretching and note any improvement in pain. Some clients are required to sleep wearing a wrist splint because movement in the night aggravates the condition. Movements of the wrist into flexion or extension may therefore be disadvantageous to such clients. However, stretching of the soft tissues around the wrist and in the forearm may help if the condition results from increased pressure in the carpal tunnel, as some studies indicate.

Active stretches

Self-tractioning of the wrist (as in figure 6.41) may be helpful.

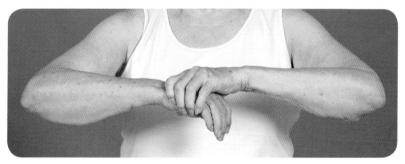

Figure 6.41

Passive stretches

Passive tractioning as shown in figure 6.37 is a gentle place to start. Stretching the palmar surface as in figure 6.42 might be helpful in easing pain, providing that the patient is able to sense the stretch and provide feedback.

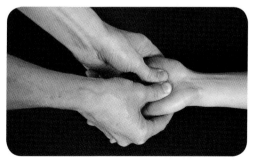

Figure 6.42

Quick Questions

1. What does swinging the arm in a pendulum-like movement do, and for which condition might it be useful?

2. What is the rationale for incorporating lateral strengthening exercises into a stretching programme for a client with tight internal rotator muscles?

3. With medial and lateral epicondylitis, why is it important to keep the elbow extended when performing stretches?

4. Why is it important to also stretch the fingers when helping someone recover from a wrist injury?

5. Which four movements of the wrist need to be regained after a sprain to this joint?

Stretching the Trunk

One of the most common complaints amongst members of the general population is lumbar pain. In this chapter you will find examples of stretches not only for the low back but also for the thorax and neck. The musculoskeletal conditions in this chapter include sub-acute whiplash, spasmodic torticollis, stiff neck, tension in neck muscles, kyphotic postures, strain of the lumbar region, and stiff lumbar spine. Altogether there are 44 stretches: 25 active and 19 passive. These are listed in table 7.1.

Note: As with the stretches provided for the conditions covered in chapters 5 and 6, the stretches in chapter 7 are not the *only* stretches that could or should be used when treating clients with back and neck conditions. Additional useful stretches for each pathology are shown in *italics* within table 7.1. The numbers in the table (e.g., 7.1, 7.2) refer to the figure numbers that illustrate the stretch. Tips plus ideas for modifying stretches are also included.

Table 7.1   Stretches for the Trunk

	Active	Passive
NECK		
Whiplash: acute	Not recommended	Not recommended
Whiplash: sub-acute	7.1, page 114 7.2, page 114 7.3, page 114 7.4, page 114	7.5, page 114
Spasmodic torticollis (wry neck)	7.6, page 115	*7.5, page 114*
Stiff neck	7.7, page 116 *7.1, page 114* *7.2, page 114* *7.3, page 114* *7.4, page 114*	7.8, page 117 7.9, page 117 7.10, page 118 7.11, page 118 7.12, page 118 7.13, page 119 7.14, page 119 7.15, page 119 7.16, page 119 *7.5, page 114*

»continued

»continued

	Active	Passive
NECK		
Tension in neck muscles	7.17, page 120 *With overpressure,* *7.1, page 114* *7.2, page 114* *7.3, page 114* *7.4, page 114* *7.6, page 115* *7.7, page 116*	*7.5, page 114* *7.8, page 117* *7.9, page 117* *7.10, page 118* *7.11, page 118* *7.12, page 118* *7.13, page 119* *7.14, page 119* *7.15, page 119* *7.16, page 119*
TRUNK		
Kyphotic postures	7.18, page 121 7.19, page 122 7.20, page 122 7.21, page 122 7.22, page 123	7.23, page 123 7.24, page 123 7.25, page 124
Low back strain: acute	Not recommended	Not recommended
Low back strain: sub-acute	7.26, page 125 7.27, page 126 7.28, page 127 7.29, page 127 7.30, page 128 7.31, page 128 7.32, page 128 7.33, page 128 7.34, page 129 7.35, page 129 7.36, page 129 *7.40, page 131*	7.37, page 130 7.38, page 130 7.39, page 130
Stiff lumbar spine	7.40, page 131 7.41, page 131 *7.26, page 125* *7.27, page 126* *7.28, page 127* *7.29, page 127* *7.30, page 128*	7.42, page 132 7.43, page 132 7.44, page 133 *7.37, page 130* *7.38, page 130* *7.39, page 130*
Herniated intervertebral disc: resolved	*With medical approval,* *7.26, page 125* *7.27, page 126* *7.28, page 127* *7.29, page 127* *7.30, page 128* *7.40, page 131* *7.41, page 131*	*With medical approval,* *7.37, page 130* *7.38, page 130* *7.39, page 130* *7.42, page 132* *7.43, page 132* *7.44, page 133*

Whiplash

Whiplash is an injury to the neck resulting from rapid acceleration or deceleration of the head or body in such a way that the neck is forced either too quickly into or past its normal range of motion. Whiplash is commonly associated with motor vehicle accidents, where the head is thrown into extension and then flexion, or thrown side to side into lateral flexion. However, the injury may occur in any other way that involves sudden jarring of the head and neck. It is characterized by pain and an unwillingness or inability to move the head due to the sudden stretching and tearing of some structures and the compression of others. The injury may result in damage to any of the structures of the neck, including muscles and their tendons, ligaments, intervertebral discs or cervical joint capsules. Blood vessels and nerves may be stretched, and in severe cases there may be fracture to cervical vertebrae.

Acute

Stretching is contraindicated in the early stages of whiplash. There is often too much pain, swelling of soft tissues and muscle spasm to make any form of stretching safe. In addition, patients may suffer dizziness and be fearful of neck movements, whether active or passive. It is important, however, for patients to return to their normal activities (including work) as soon as possible (providing these are deemed safe) in order to lessen the likelihood of the condition becoming chronic. It is therefore essential for therapists to liaise with medical practitioners in order to determine the earliest safe time for intervention.

Sub-Acute

It is important to maintain and improve range of motion (ROM) as soon as possible. Where therapeutic intervention is delayed, patients sometimes develop wry neck (see page 115). It is difficult to define the sub-acute stage precisely, although this could be when pain subsides. In most cases performing the gentle ROM stretches illustrated here will be beneficial for recovery from whiplash. However, if clients experience pain, numbness, tingling or dizziness whilst performing any of these movements, they should stop.

Active stretches

Sometimes patients with whiplash are immobilized in a soft collar that when removed leaves the patients feeling vulnerable and unwilling to move the head and neck normally for fear of reinjury. As a result tissues of the neck may shorten, leading to impairment not only of the neck but possibly of the shoulder too. It is therefore important to regain normal range of motion in the neck as soon as possible. Simple range of motion exercises are a safe yet often underused means of stretching. Instruct your client to *slowly* perform flexion (figure 7.1), extension (figure 7.2), lateral flexion (figure 7.3) and rotation (figure 7.4) at regular intervals throughout the day. Flexion helps stretch the neck extensors (such as the erector spinae and upper fibres of the trapezius); extension helps stretch the neck flexors (such as the scalenes); lateral flexion and rotation help stretch the upper fibres of the trapezius and sternocleidomastoid on the side away from which the head is moved. For best effect, the client should keep the shoulders facing forwards and avoid bending to one side or rotating with the trunk.

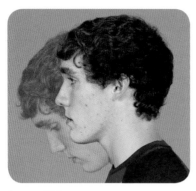

Figure 7.1

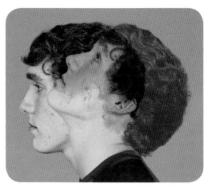

Figure 7.2

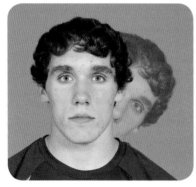

Figure 7.3

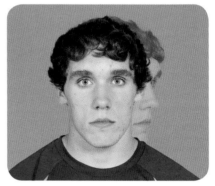

Figure 7.4

TIP If a client finds it uncomfortable to perform these stretches seated with her hands resting in her lap, have her rest her forearms and elbows on the arms of a chair such that the shoulders are ever so slightly passively elevated. In this position, there is slightly less tension in muscles that elevate the shoulder (levator scapulae and upper fibres of the trapezius) and the associated fascia, making active neck stretches more comfortable.

Passive stretches

A safe and gentle passive stretch is to facilitate neck rotation using a towel, which minimizes tension on the tissues. Position the towel beneath the patient's head, and gently move the towel to bring about passive rotation (figure 7.5).

TIP If a client can feel the treatment couch beneath his head, he feels supported and is more likely to relax than if he cannot feel the couch. Lifting the head is therefore not necessary and may in fact be disadvantageous.

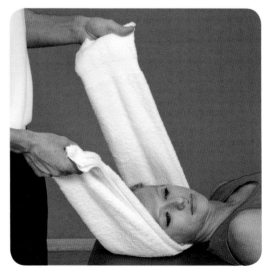

Figure 7.5

Spasmodic Torticollis (Wry Neck)

There are several types of torticollis, or wry neck. Spasmodic torticollis is sometimes experienced by clients who have suffered previous injury to the neck, including whiplash, and involves painful spasming of the sternocleidomastoid, upper fibres of the trapezius or both.

Active stretches

Clients suffering from spasmodic torticollis find active neck movements difficult and painful. They may find it helpful to rest in the position shown in figure 7.6, turning their head *away* from the side they feel the spasm. This position helps stretch the muscles that are spasming and also gently tractions the neck extensors if a small pillow or support is used as shown. Encourage your clients to take their time getting into this position, relaxing in order to lower muscle tone, decreasing the spasm.

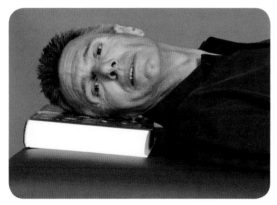

Figure 7.6

Passive stretches

Gentle passive movement using a towel as in figure 7.5 is helpful. However, it is important to remember that muscles are prone to cramping when held in a shortened position, so be cautious when turning the head towards the side of the spasm.

Stiff Neck

There are many causes of a stiff neck. Some of the musculoskeletal causes include maintaining a static position for too long, as when engaged in a long telephone conversation or working at a computer. Sports involving overarm movements, such as tennis, badminton, rock climbing or swimming, may lead to soreness and tension in neck muscles and a sensation of 'pulling' when the head is turned one way. Some clients report that their necks feel stiff if they sit or stand in a draft or sleep awkwardly. Patients who have suffered whiplash often experience a decrease in cervical ROM accompanied by feelings of neck stiffness if they have not addressed ROM as part of their rehabilitation. In each of these examples, stretching can be beneficial in decreasing muscular tension and reducing feelings of stiffness.

Active stretches

Active stretches are an important part of self-management for patients with a stiff neck. A good start is to suggest the ROM stretches shown in the section for sub-acute whiplash (figures 7.1 through 7.4).

TIP One way to encourage clients to decrease stiffness by performing cervical rotation is to suggest that each time they look over their shoulder, they try to see farther behind themselves, noting what they can observe. Also, rotation with overpressure is sometimes easier for clients to perform if they do this stretch in the supine position.

Active cervical ROM movements can be modified by suggesting the client add gentle overpressure, for example, as he performs lateral neck flexion (figure 7.7). In this example, depressing the shoulder (by reaching down towards the floor) helps to further stretch the lateral neck flexors because some of these muscles (levator scapulae and upper fibres of the trapezius) are also shoulder elevators.

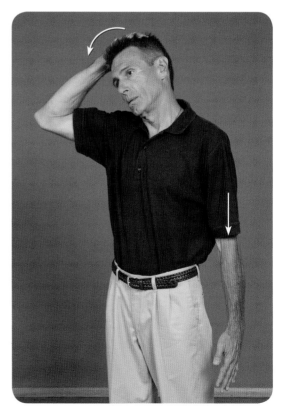

Figure 7.7

Passive stretches

Gentle passive rotation of the neck using a towel (figure 7.5) is a useful starting point when treating clients with a stiff neck. If you are reading this as a massage therapist, you may be used to applying gentle soft tissue tractioning to the cervical extensors as shown in figure 7.8. With a small amount of lubricant, you can gently draw your fingertips up the client's neck, on either side of the spinous processes, gently pulling into the skin and underlying soft tissues. Gentle sustained pressure into the occipital bone will facilitate creep in tissues and may help improve forward flexion of the neck. Try this seated or kneeling to see which position works best for you as a therapist.

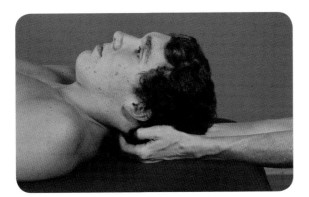

Figure 7.8

An alternative is to apply gentle traction using a towel as shown in figure 7.9. Hook the towel gently against the occipital bone, and keeping the towel close to the client's head, apply sustained traction for about 30 seconds. Avoid extending the neck.

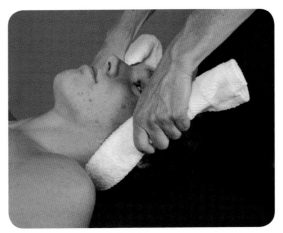

Figure 7.9

Three other passive stretches are useful. These are for the lateral neck flexors and are each easily modified to become MET stretches. With the client supine, you could passively stretch the lateral neck flexors by gently depressing the shoulder and simultaneously easing the head and neck into lateral flexion (figure 7.10). This stretch can also be performed with the client seated (figure 7.11).

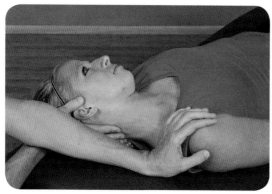

Figure 7.10

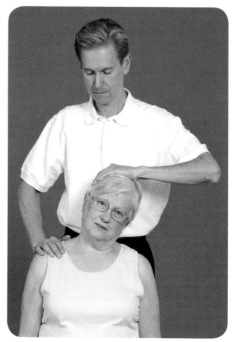

Figure 7.11

Or, both shoulders can be depressed simultaneously (figure 7.12), helping to stretch the shoulder elevator muscles.

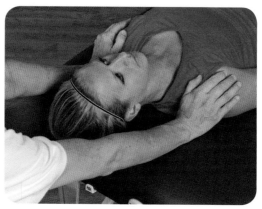

Figure 7.12

Soft tissue release is another useful type of stretching for treating stiff necks and may be performed to the trapezius (figures 7.13 and 7.14) or more specifically to the levator scapulae (figures 7.15 and 7.16).

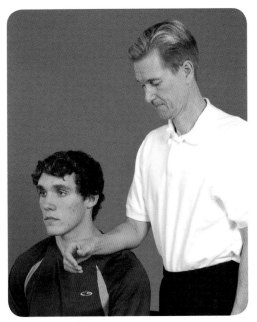

Figure 7.13

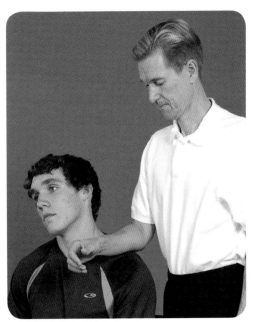

Figure 7.14

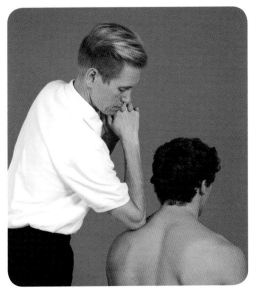

Figure 7.15

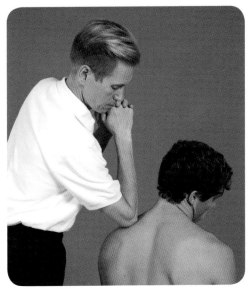

Figure 7.16

Tension in Neck Muscles

Tension develops in neck muscles in much the same way as stiffness occurs in this region: lack of movement, sustaining static positions for long periods of time or excessive use of shoulder and neck muscles. In addition, tension increases when we are feeling anxious or stressed. All the stretches illustrated so far, both active and passive, are helpful in addressing tension in neck muscles.

Active stretches

In addition to figures 7.1 through 7.4, 7.6 and 7.7, simple retraction of the head (figure 7.17) helps stretch out the small intervertebral muscles on the posterior of the neck. Note that this is quite different from extending the head and neck as shown in figure 7.2. In figure 7.17 the client is asked to imagine that his chin is resting on a shelf, drawing it back to give himself the appearance of a 'double' chin. This movement may be practised regularly throughout the day and helps stretch tissues of the cervical region quite differently from neck extension, which compresses (rather than stretches) tissues of the posterior neck. Many clients dislike the sensation of this stretch because it stretches some tissues and compresses others that are not normally affected in this way. It is, however, an especially important stretch to include for treating clients with increased cervical lordosis.

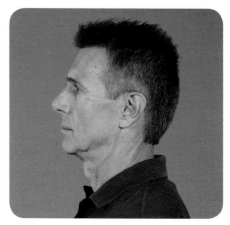

Figure 7.17

TIP A good way to be sure your client is performing this simple stretch correctly is to ask her to lie supine. Place your finger in the lordotic curve of her neck, around the middle vertebra of this region, and request that she try to push her neck into your finger, backwards and into the couch. As she attempts this, gently draw your finger from her neck to the couch so that she is forced to perform a retraction-type movement in order for her neck to maintain contact with your finger.

Passive stretches

All the passive stretches in figures 7.5 through 7.16 are useful when treating people with tension in the neck muscles.

Kyphotic Postures

Kyphosis is an increase in the normal outward curvature of the spine, often due to thoracic vertebrae becoming anteriorly reduced and wedge shaped in elderly people. However, many younger people develop kyphotic postures as the result of sitting for long periods of time in a slumped position so that muscles of the anterior part of the body shorten and those of the posterior part of the body lengthen, producing an imbalance in forces acting on the vertebral column and a curvature in response to tension in anterior muscles. With kyphotic postures the scapulae protract, bringing with them the humeri, which may fall into internal rotation. It is therefore important to check for and address any shortening of muscles associated with this posture. (For information on stretching the internal rotators of the humerus, see page 95 in chapter 6, Stretching the Upper Limb). Both active and passive stretches are helpful in lengthening pectoral muscles.

Active stretches

There are many ways to actively stretch the pectorals. Five examples are shown here. In figure 7.18, the client simply stands with his arm against a wall or door frame and takes a small step forward until he feels the stretch in his chest and anterior shoulder region. Moving the hand upwards from the horizontal position stretches different fibres of the pectoralis major muscle.

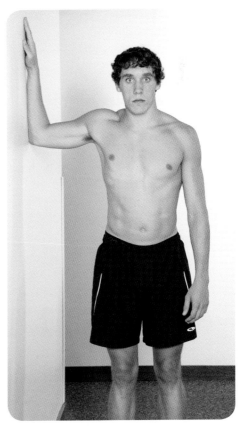

Figure 7.18

By contrast, a more advanced stretch is that shown in figure 7.19. Here the client needs to be able to safely position herself onto (and off of) a gym ball and rest as shown. These positions may be unsuitable for some clients, such as the elderly or someone unable to stand or lacking balance.

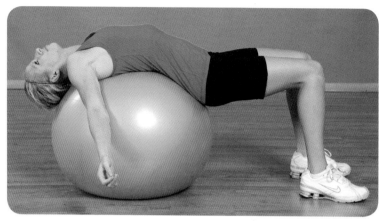

Figure 7.19

Alternatives include simply resting in the supine position with a bolster, pillow or rolled-up towel lengthwise along the thorax and head as in figure 7.20.

Remember that simply contracting the rhomboid muscles by drawing the scapulae together (figure 7.21) inhibits contraction in the pectorals. This exercise could be repeated at regular intervals throughout the day, especially for people who spend long periods of time in a seated position.

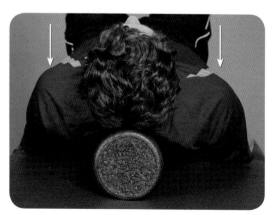

Figure 7.20

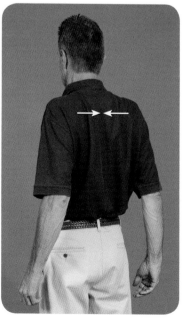

Figure 7.21

Last, a client could use a towel as shown in figure 7.22, either whilst seated or standing. Such a stretch is good for clients unable to clasp their hands together behind their backs.

Passive stretches

One of the simplest ways to stretch the pectorals passively is to position your client supine on a therapy couch and apply pressure to the shoulders as shown in figure 7.23. To increase the stretch, you could position the client on a bolster or rolled-up towel, placed lengthwise down the thoracic region, taking care to also support the head.

The pectorals may also be stretched unilaterally—that is, one side of the body at a time, as in figure 7.24. This is helpful where a client is unable to tolerate a bilateral stretch, perhaps because of a shoulder injury on one side, making stretching of that side contraindicated. To stretch one side of the chest and armpit, it is necessary to position the client with the arm stretched so that the shoulder sits on the edge of the treatment couch. This enables you to gently ease the arm into horizontal extension. Another advantage of performing a pectoral stretch in this way is that it facilitates leverage and is helpful when stretching very strong clients.

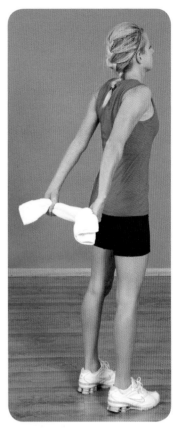

Figure 7.22

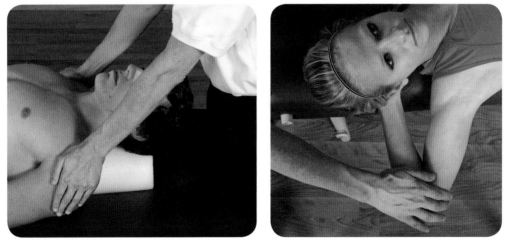

Figure 7.23

Figure 7.24

TIP When performing the unilateral stretch, it is better not to use the bolster because the client tends to roll off of it as you depress one side of the client's body.

An alternative bilateral pectoral stretch is to stand behind a seated client and gently ease back her arms as shown in figure 7.25. Keep the client sitting upright, perhaps by placing a pillow or bolster down her back to prevent hyperextension of the spine. Holding the client in this position is useful if the client is stronger than you because you may use *your* shoulder adductor muscles to help bring about the stretch on your client. The disadvantage is that you cannot see the client and must take care to let her guide you in where to start the stretch.

Both stretches 7.24 and 7.25 can be used as starting positions for MET stretches.

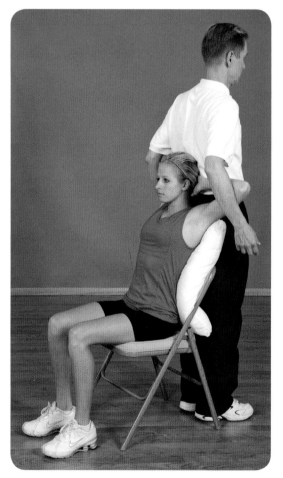

Figure 7.25

Low Back Strain

Strain of the muscles of the low back is a common injury, usually occurring in movements such as unsupported forward or lateral flexion whilst a person is moving a heavy object. In many cases strain occurs because of physical fatigue of muscles or injury from sporting activities, especially those involving twisting movements with or without lateral flexion. The very deep quadratus lumborum or the more superficial muscles of the erector spinae group may be injured. Muscle soreness at the site of injury may occur, along with spasming of muscles above or below this. Without stretching, the tissues may shorten and the region may feel stiff, with loss of range in motion. Yet stretching too soon after the initial injury risks damaging unhealed structures and delaying the rehabilitation process.

Acute

Both active and passive stretches are contraindicated in the acute stages of back strain. Care is needed to confirm that only muscle and fascia are damaged and not more serious structures such as an intervertebral disc or facet joints, for example.

Sub-Acute

Your aim at this stage might be to decrease spasming in muscles such as the quadratus lumborum and the erector spinae and maintain range of motion in the lumbar region. Usually, the absence of pain is a good indication that it is safe to start a programme of gentle stretches.

Active stretches

There are many useful stretches clients may perform themselves to combat the problems associated with sub-acute strain of the lumbar spine. A good starting point is for a client to rest in a position that will gently traction the extensor muscles and associated fascia (figure 7.26).

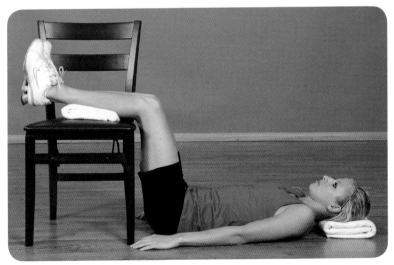

Figure 7.26

To improve lumbar movement, simple hip hitching is useful to stretch the soft tissues of this area before weight bearing can be tolerated. The client lies in a neutral position (figure 7.27a) and, keeping his torso still, tries to draw up his hip first on one side (figure 7.27b) and then on the other (figure 7.27c). The effect is to facilitate lateral flexion of the trunk whilst supine, eliminating the effects of gravity on this stretch.

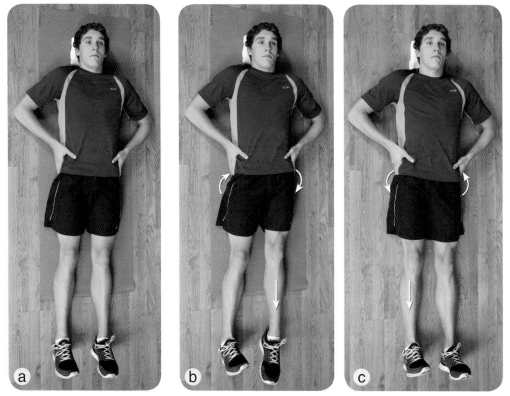

Figure 7.27

Still in the supine position, the client could practise pelvic tilting, gently tilting her pelvis into the posterior tilt position, flattening her back against the bed (figure 7.28) or hugging one or both legs (figure 7.29). Both actions help stretch the lumbar extensors, thus facilitating lumbar flexion.

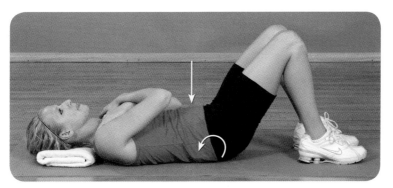

Figure 7.28

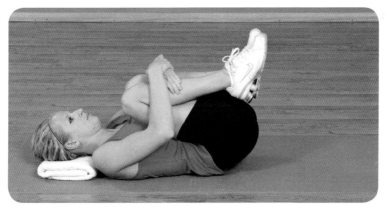

Figure 7.29

Once stretches are well tolerated in the supine position, the client could progress to seated stretches. These could include hugging one knee at a time (figure 7.30) or forward flexion (figure 7.31), both of which help stretch lumbar extensors, with 7.31 being the greater stretch.

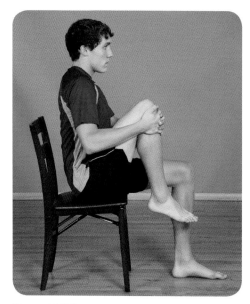

Figure 7.30

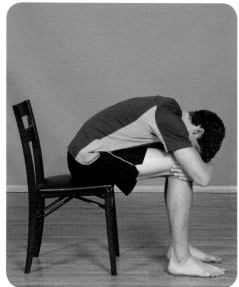

Figure 7.31

Rotation of the spine can be added (figure 7.32) as well as lateral flexion (figure 7.33). Note that it is better for a client to perform active rotation of the trunk in a seated position rather than standing because in standing clients have a tendency to rotate from the feet, ankles and hips rather than the waist and therefore do not get a proper low back stretch.

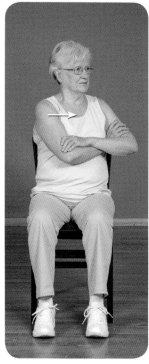

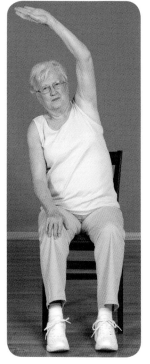

Figure 7.32

Figure 7.33

After seated stretches, the client could progress to standing stretches. Remember that all your stretches may be modified to suit each client's needs and abilities. For some, simply resting in a semi-flexed position with support (figure 7.34) will be enough to stretch the extensor muscles and fascia of the lumbar area. Eventually the client may need to facilitate an increase in ROM of the lumbar spine by practising pelvic tilting in the upright position. As with the same stretch performed in the supine position, the posterior pelvic tilt (figure 7.35) stretches the extensors, and this could be alternated with an anterior pelvic tilt (figure 7.36).

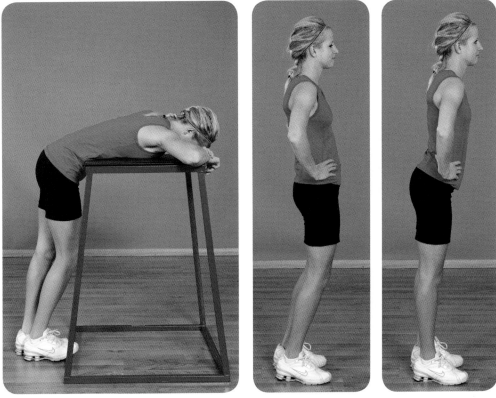

Figure 7.34   Figure 7.35   Figure 7.36

 Clients instructed to perform rotation in the standing position have a tendency to turn their entire bodies rather than just the torso. It is therefore better to perform rotatory movements either sitting (as in figure 7.32) or, if the client can tolerate it, as in figure 7.40, found in the next section on stretches for a stiff lumbar spine. Lateral flexion is also quite strenuous to perform in the standing position. Lateral flexion to the right, for example, necessitates eccentric contraction of the left quadratus lumborum in order to hold the body in this position against gravity.

Passive stretches

The main focus of passive stretching should be to regain normal range of motion in the lumbar region. Three ways to gently stretch the lumbar extensor muscles are to ease the client into a position of hip and knee flexion whilst supine (figure 7.37), to gently traction the lower limbs (figure 7.38) and to place a towel beneath the thoracic and lumbar areas and gently tug it out from between the client's legs (figure 7.39). Although this last manoeuvre seems a little unorthodox, it has the effect of passively moving the lumbar spine into a position of decreased lordosis by posteriorly tilting the pelvis.

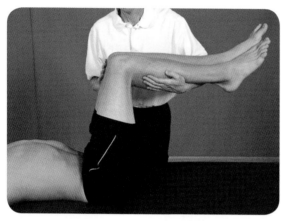

Figure 7.37

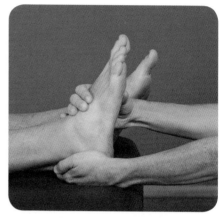

Figure 7.38

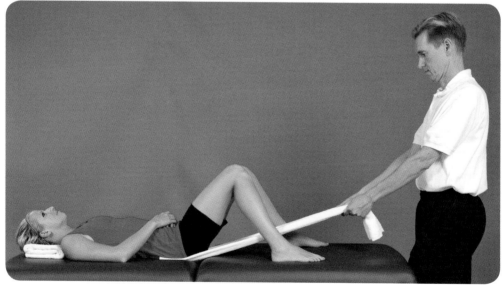

Figure 7.39

Stiff Lumbar Spine

The lumbar region may become stiff for reasons similar to those causing stiffness in other regions of the spine, namely immobility or after injury. Many of the active and passive stretches in the section on sub-acute low back strain may be helpful. Additional stretches may be useful, and these are described below.

Active stretches

In addition to the stretches shown in the section for sub-acute low back strain (figures 7.26 through 7.30), clients may benefit from this supine rotatory stretch (figure 7.40) and this seated rotatory stretch (figure 7.41), using the upper limb to increase the stretch in each example.

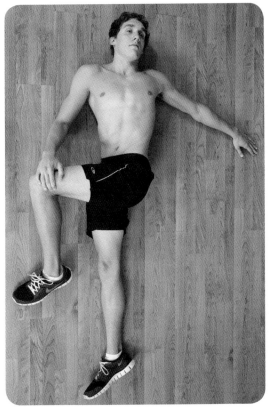

Figure 7.40

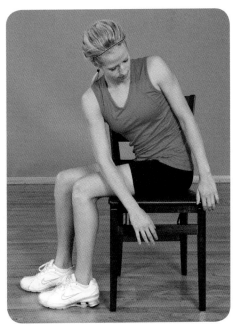

Figure 7.41

Passive stretches

Popular methods of stretching the soft tissues of the lumbar area, especially quadratus lumborum, are to apply gentle overpressure to the client as she rests in a position of rotation whilst supine (figure 7.42) or, more dramatically, in a side-lying position, sometimes with a small towel beneath the waist (figure 7.43). To increase the stretch further, the client could be positioned, with caution, on a gym ball (figure 7.44). Not all clients with a stiff low back will feel comfortable in these positions, and such clients may need to emphasize active stretches in their programmes.

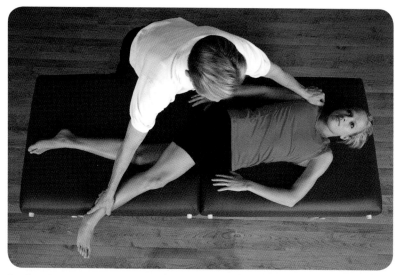

Figure 7.42

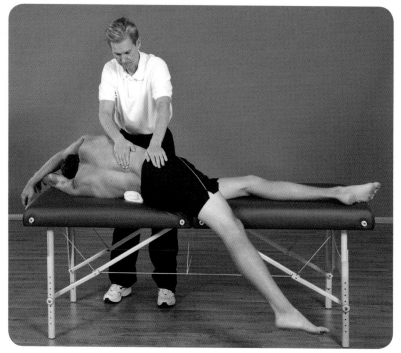

Figure 7.43

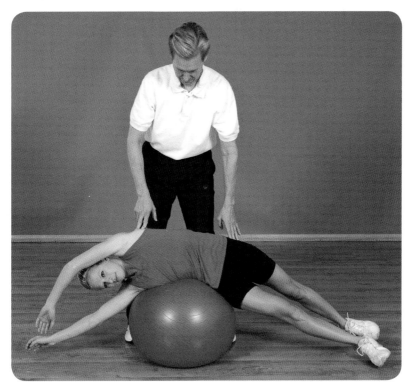

Figure 7.44

In addition, clients may benefit from the passive stretches shown in the section for sub-acute low back strain (figures 7.37 through 7.39).

Herniated Intervertebral Disc

Herniation of an intervertebral disc (popularly known as a 'slipped' disc) is common. However, stretching is totally contraindicated in the acute condition and potentially dangerous in the sub-acute condition. As with many conditions affecting the lumbar spine, keeping the region mobile rather than immobile is preferable. However, in the initial stages of repair, clients recovering from disc herniations should be encouraged to rest and to move only within their pain-free range. Movements to encourage mobility are introduced gradually by a physical therapist or similarly trained professional.

Perhaps because of the severity of the pain, or lack of advice from a medical professional, many clients avoid movement entirely and as a consequence are left with severe stiffness and decreased ROM in the lumbar region. When the condition has resolved, whether naturally or as a result of surgical intervention, stiffness in the lumbar region may be a significant limiting factor for these clients. Such clients are therefore likely to benefit from gentle stretches, such as many of those illustrated for low back strain (see page 125, particularly figures 7.26 through 7.30) and stiff lumbar spine (see page 131, figures 7.40 and 7.41), providing you have medical approval.

Quick Questions

1. Why is it better if a client can feel the treatment couch beneath his head when receiving passive neck rotations using a towel?

2. What verbal tip could you give to your client to encourage her to perform the movement of head and neck retraction correctly?

3. Which simple exercise could a client perform during the day to help relax the pectoral muscles?

4. When treating a client for low back strain, should the movements of hip hitching be used before or after the client is able to bear weight?

5. Why might it be better for a client to perform active rotation of the trunk in a seated position rather than a standing position?

PART IV

Stretching Routines

In this final part of *Therapeutic Stretching*, you will find a visual guide to passive stretching routines that can be performed in the prone (chapter 8), supine (chapter 9) and seated (chapter 10) positions. These routines help you practise the stretches—perhaps using a family member, friend or colleague—so you can incorporate them into your practice without having to ask a client to constantly change position in order to receive a particular stretch. Of course, in reality, you would not necessarily perform an entire series of stretches in any one position when using therapeutic stretching on a client recovering from a musculoskeletal condition. Instead, you would concentrate on one particular body part rather than one particular treatment position. Nevertheless, it may sometimes be necessary to provide stretches in one position (e.g., if a client were bedbound or suffering from more than one condition).

Accompanying each photograph (selected from earlier chapters), you will find a reminder of key points. Use each treatment position to help you practise some of the stretches provided in chapters 5, 6 and 7, but remember that these routines are not set in stone. They are provided as a guide only to help you become familiar with how you might apply the stretches, and they will be particularly helpful if you are new to passive stretching. Questions at the end of chapter 10 will help you reflect on your performance. They have no right or wrong answers.

8

Prone Stretching Routine

Six prone stretches are featured in this chapter, four for the lower limb and two for the upper limb. For practising the six stretches in this sequence, it will be helpful to have a small towel or firm sponge on hand to position beneath your subject's knee when performing the stretch to the rectus femoris. Note: There are no passive stretches for the trunk in prone. Most of the conditions affecting the spine for which therapeutic stretching might be appropriate are performed in either the supine or seated positions (and sometimes even in side-lying).

Calf Stretch

Remember that for this stretch, your client needs to have his feet positioned off the edge of the treatment couch as shown.

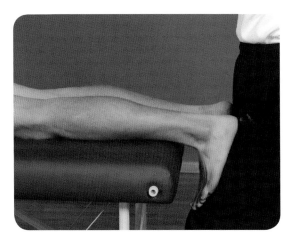

Quadriceps Stretch

Remember to stabilize the pelvis by leaning on the sacrum. This is particularly important when treating clients with very tight quadriceps because the rectus femoris will tend to tilt the pelvis anteriorly during the stretch if the pelvis is not stabilized in this way.

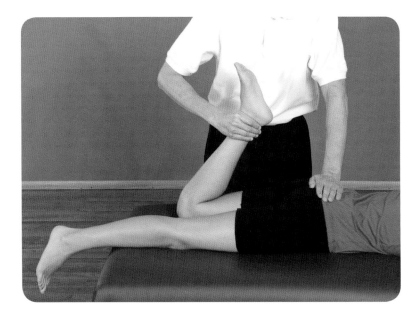

Soleus Stretch

If you recall from chapter 5, this stretch is not appropriate for clients who have conditions affecting the knee on the side of the calf that is being stretched.

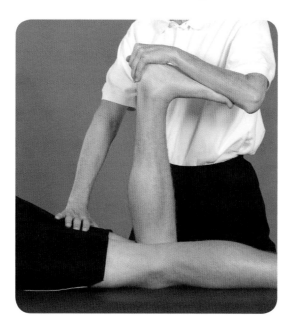

Rectus Femoris Stretch

Notice that by positioning the towel as shown, the hip is taken into extension, thus increasing the stretch on the hip flexors (particularly rectus femoris) rather than the quadriceps.

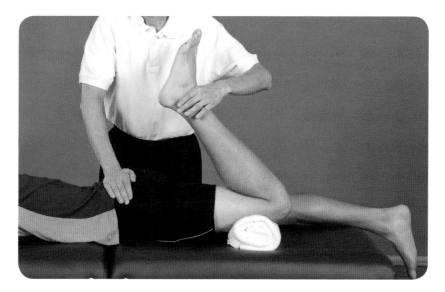

Shoulder Traction

Notice that in this picture, the therapist is supporting the client's arm, avoiding traction to the elbow joint.

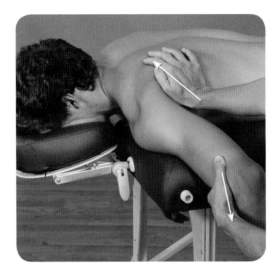

Supraspinatus Stretch

If you are having difficulty locating the supraspinatus, ask your subject to abduct her arm, and you should feel this muscle contract.

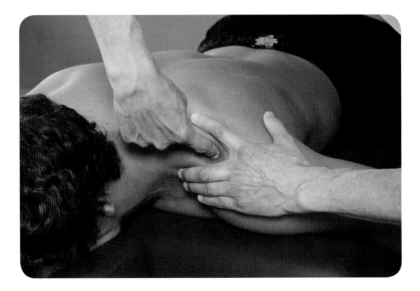

9

Supine
Stretching Routine

This chapter features 34 supine stretches: 12 for the lower limb, 11 for the upper limb and 11 for the trunk. For practising the stretches in this sequence, you will need a small towel to position beneath your client's head for the neck stretches and the passive posterior pelvic tilt, and perhaps a bolster or rolled-up towel for the bilateral pectoral stretch.

Calf Stretch

This position requires considerable leverage. Compare this to stretching the calf whilst prone.

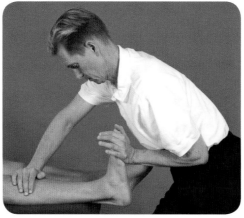

Toe Flexor Stretch

If your client is particularly ticklish, try applying this stretch through a towel.

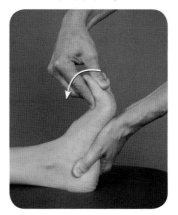

Tibialis Anterior Stretch

Remember that our feet naturally fall into plantar flexion at rest, and overstretching the anterior aspect could increase the likelihood of ankle sprains, so use this stretch only when treating clients with particularly stiff ankles.

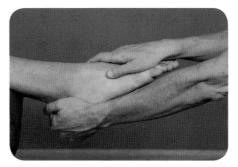

Ankle Traction

Remember that this stretch tractions not only the ankle but the knee and hip, too.

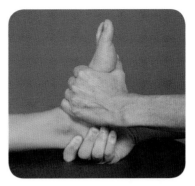

STR to Tibialis Anterior

Use the information provided in chapter 5 (page 64) to help you practise STR to the tibialis anterior.

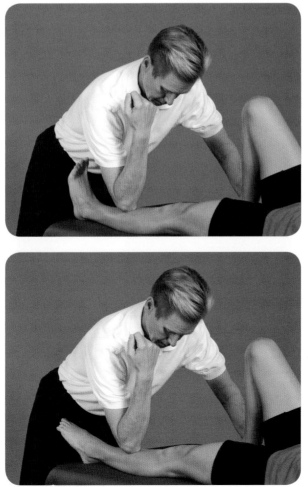

Passive Knee Flexion and Extension

When practising this movement, keep the client's lower limb close to your own body so you do not need to lean across the treatment couch. The legs are heavy, and you need to avoid straining your low back when applying passive stretches to the limb in this way.

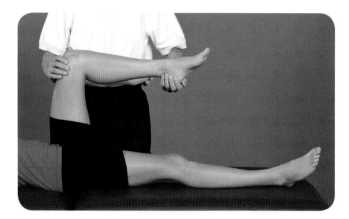

Passive Straight-Leg Hamstring Stretch

Whilst this stretch is shown in the supine position, it can be tricky to apply it with the client on a treatment couch. Practise applying this stretch with the client on a couch or on the floor, as shown here. Remember to safeguard your own posture when applying this stretch.

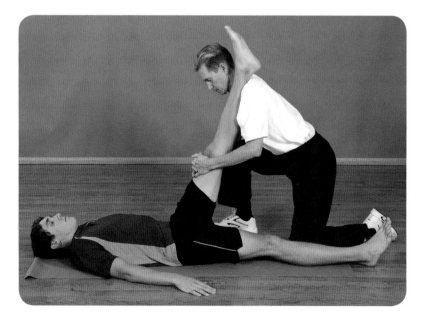

Flexed-Knee Adductor Stretch

Remember to prevent the client's pelvis from tilting by gently placing your hand over the anterior superior iliac spine as shown.

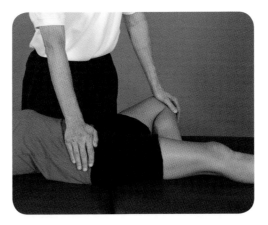

Straight-Leg Adductor Stretch

Notice how this tensions soft tissues on the medial side of the knee. Which of these two stretches does your client prefer to receive, this one or the previous one?

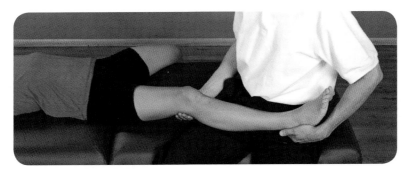

Quadriceps Stretch

This is a good way to stretch the quadriceps and rectus femoris, particularly in clients who are comfortable in this treatment position. Try kneeling to apply the stretch rather than bending over to hold the client's ankle to flex the knee.

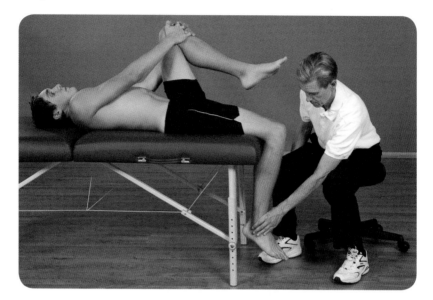

Hip Flexors Stretch

Again, your client needs to be comfortable in this position for this to be an effective stretch.

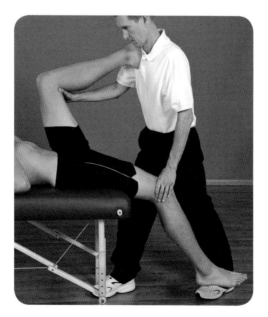

Gluteals Stretch

As with the hamstrings, performing passive gluteal stretches is useful but can be difficult on a treatment couch. Compare how easy (or not) it is to stretch the gluteals, first with your client on a treatment couch and then on the floor.

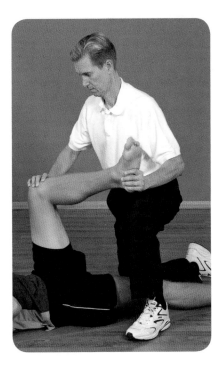

Gentle Shoulder Traction

Notice how the therapist is tractioning the shoulder rather than the whole of the upper limb.

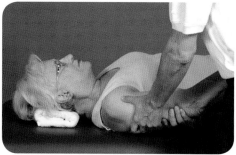

Gentle Shoulder Traction With Lateral Neck Flexion

Remember, the key to this stretch is for you as a therapist to *apply the gentle traction first* and then for the client to laterally flex. Performing the stretch this way means the client is in charge of how much tension is or is not directed at the soft tissues of the shoulder and neck.

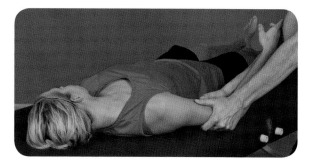

Shoulder Traction With Flexion

Practise gently lifting your client in this manner, taking care not to pinch the elbow by gripping too hard. Notice how heavy the arms are. Keep the client close to you in order to avoid straining your back as you gently traction the shoulder at 90 degrees of flexion as shown.

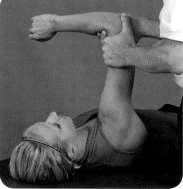

Anterior Shoulder Stretch

Practise positioning your hands in various places on your subject's shoulder, and get feedback to help you determine in which position she feels the most stretch.

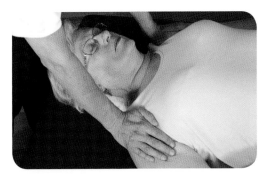

Stretch of Internal Rotators

For this stretch, the client does not need to have the shoulder abducted to 90 degrees. This is a good stretch position from which to apply MET. Look back at the MET section in chapter 4, and gently apply MET if you are practising on a client with tight internal rotators.

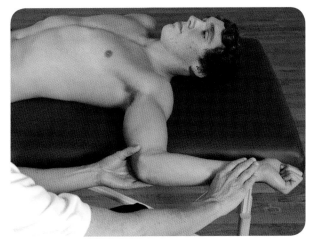

Passive Flexion (and Extension) of the Elbow

As with flexion and extension of the wrist, practise applying these to your client in both the supine and seated positions.

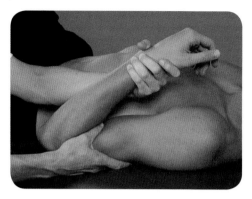

Wrist Flexion (and Extension)

It is a good idea to try flexion and extension stretches with your client in the supine position. Compare how easy (or not) it is to apply these stretches compared to performing them with your client seated.

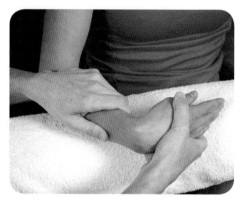

Gentle Ulnar (and Radial) Deviation

Practise various handholds to identify which feels most comfortable for both you and your client.

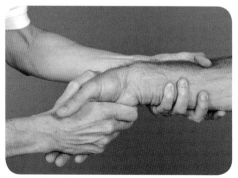

Gentle Wrist Traction

The wrist can be tractioned in the supine and prone positions. In the supine position, you also have the ability to stretch the palmar surface (the next stretch) as well as extend and stretch the fingers.

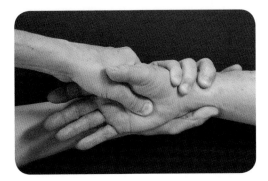

Stretching the Palmar Surface

Keep your client's elbow (flexed) resting on the treatment couch when you work on the wrist and fingers.

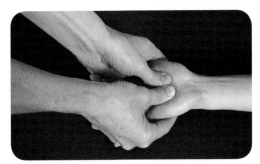

Stretching the Fingers

When practising this stretch, notice how it is increased if you *also* extend the wrist.

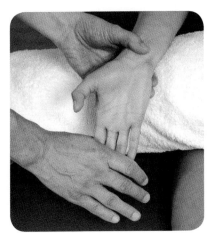

Gentle Neck Stretches

Remember to keep the client's head against the treatment couch when you practise this stretch.

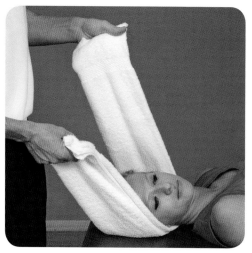

Stretching Sub-Occipital Muscles

Sitting to apply this stretch prevents you from having to flex too much at the waist.

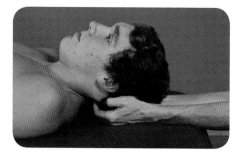

Gentle Towel Stretch

Practising on family and friends is a good way to investigate where to position the towel and in which direction to pull in order to get the best gentle neck stretch for your client.

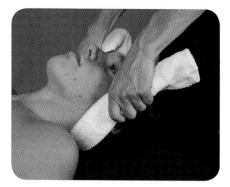

Unilateral Trapezius Stretch

This (and the stretch that follows) is a good starting position from which to begin an MET stretch. Look back at chapter 4 to discover how to do this form of stretching.

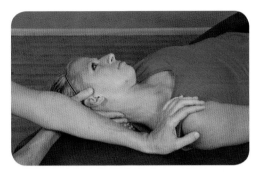

Bilateral Trapezius Stretch

Asking your client to exhale as you gently depress the shoulders helps facilitate relaxation in the often-tight upper section of the trapezius.

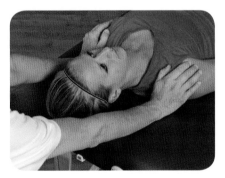

Bilateral Pectoral Stretch

Remember that using a rolled-up towel or bolster longitudinally placed beneath the thoracic spine (and supporting the head) will greatly increase the sensation of stretch when pressure is applied to the shoulders in this manner.

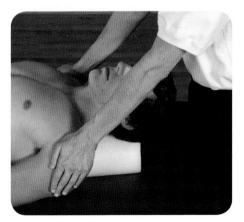

Unilateral Pectoral Stretch

Be certain to position your client with her shoulder on the edge of the treatment couch in order to allow for horizontal extension during this stretch.

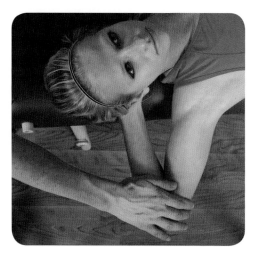

Passive Lumbar Flexion

Keep the client close to you when holding his legs in this way in order to avoid straining your own back.

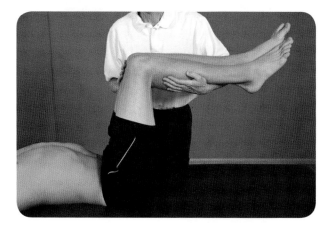

Unilateral Lower Limb Traction

Remember that this tractions not only the lumbar spine but the hips, knees and ankles too.

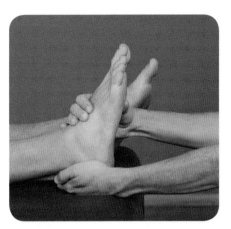

Passive Posterior Pelvic Tilt

Using a towel to help your client experience passive posterior tilt helps stretch the extensors of the lumbar spine.

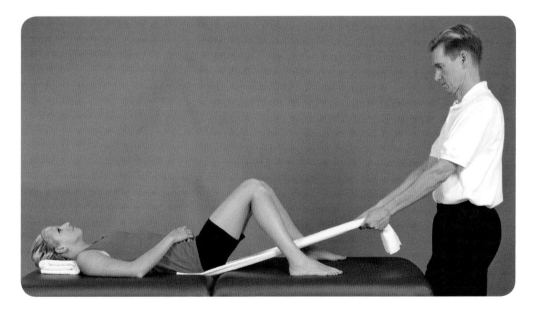

Passive Quadratus Lumborum Stretch

Compare how it feels to perform this stretch with your subject on a treatment couch to what it is like to apply it on the floor.

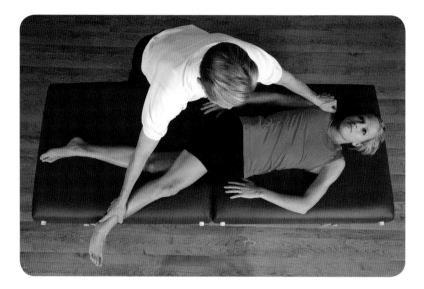

Seated Stretching Routine

This chapter features 15 seated stretches: 2 for the lower limb, 9 for the upper limb and 4 for the trunk. These stretches are selected from chapters 5, 6 and 7. It does not matter in which order you practise them. That is, you could choose to start on the trunk and practise those stretches, and then move to the upper limb and then to the lower limb. You could practise them with your client seated on a chair or on the edge of a treatment couch. Experiment with whether your subject needs a back rest for support.

Foot and Ankle Stretch

The feet and ankles may be stretched with the client supine or seated. In the supine position, you have the advantage of being able to position the client's feet at a suitable height for your treatment. In the seated position, you have less flexibility but can still perform stretches by having your client rest his feet on a stool, a chair or even your lap. In the seated position it is also possible to apply a calf stretch. In addition to the stretch shown here, refer to stretches 5.5 and 5.6 (page 57), and consider how these might be peformed with your client seated.

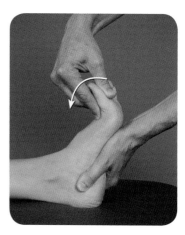

Knee and Thigh Stretch

It is also possible to stretch the hamstrings and quadriceps when your client is in the seated position. Of course, this is only applicable for treating clients with restrictions in knee ROM as a result of tension in these muscles, or for treating clients unable to rest comfortably in either the prone or supine position. For clients with good flexibility, seated stretches are not appropriate because in this position the knee cannot be fully flexed. For clients with tension in the posterior capsule of the knee, seated hamstring stretches may be useful. Consider the comfort of your client and whether she needs a back support whilst seated.

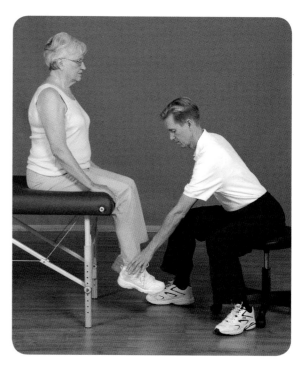

Gentle Shoulder Traction

Compare how it feels to apply this stretch to a client in the seated position with how it feels to apply it with the client supine. In the previous section you practised gentle shoulder traction combined with lateral neck flexion. How might that work in the seated position?

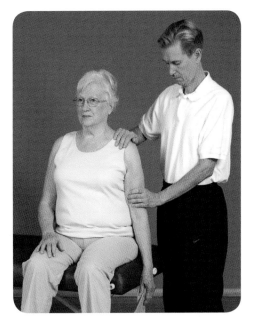

Stretching Internal Shoulder Rotators

Holding your client's arm as shown and gently taking the humerus into lateral rotation stretches the internal rotators. Compare this to the same stretch with the client supine. Can you see how in the seated position the stretch is different because the arm is adducted, whereas in the supine position the arm is abducted?

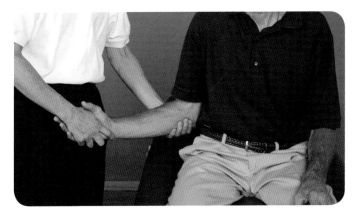

Gentle Elbow Stretches

Holding the forearm and elbow as shown is a good way to stretch the muscles of pronation and supination. Elbow flexion and extension can also be easily performed in the seated position.

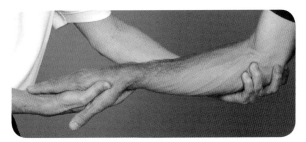

Gentle Wrist Flexion

Compare how it feels to passively stretch the extensors, flexors and muscles of ulnar and radial deviation with a client seated and in the supine position.

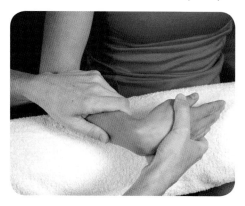

Gentle Wrist Extension

Notice that by also taking the fingers into extension, the client experiences a greater stretch.

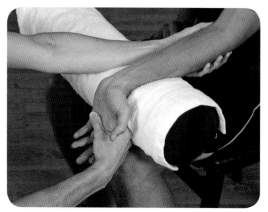

Ulnar (and Radial) Deviation

Be cautious with this stretch, because there is far less movement in the wrist in these ranges of movement compared with flexion and extension.

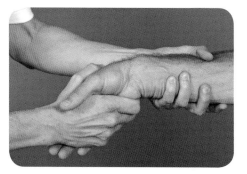

Gentle Wrist Traction

Which handhold works best for you and your client when applying gentle traction to the wrist?

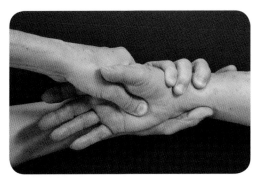

Stretching Finger Flexors

Notice that the sensation of stretch in the finger flexors is increased when the elbow is extended in addition to the wrist and fingers.

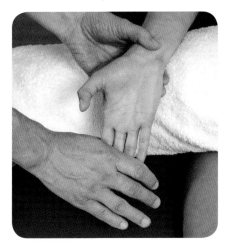

Stretching the Palm

Experiment with which handhold works best for you as you try to spread the metacarpal heads of the hand.

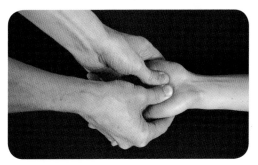

Gentle Neck Stretch

Remember to apply this stretch cautiously, getting feedback from your subject as you do.

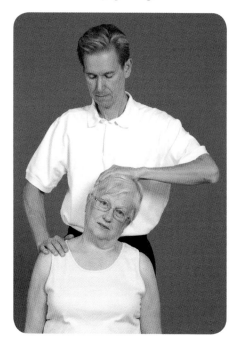

STR to Trapezius

Soft tissue release to the upper fibres of the trapezius or levator scapulae is easy to apply with your client in the seated position. Refer to chapter 4 for guidance on performing this advanced form of stretching.

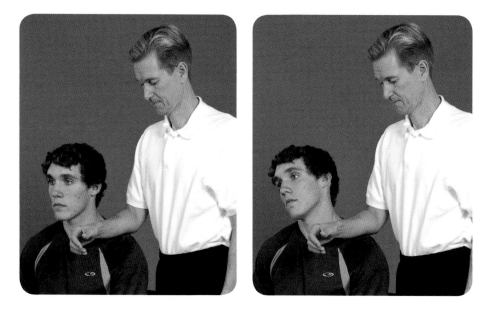

STR to Levator Scapulae

Remember that using an elbow localizes your pressure, but this does not mean you should add more force. All these passive stretches should be pain free.

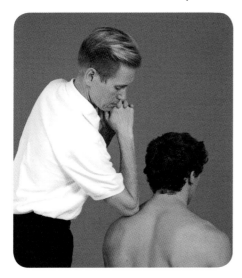 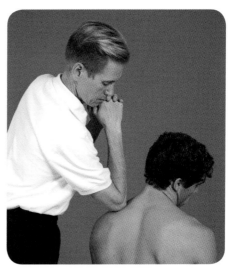

Seated Pectoral Stretch

Sometimes it helps to place a pillow or bolster (longitudinally) at your client's back to avoid extending her spine as you gently draw her shoulders back. Remember to get feedback because it is easy to overstretch people in this position. Remember, too, that you do not need to stand back to back as shown here; you could turn around so you are facing your client's back before you gently draw her arms into extension.

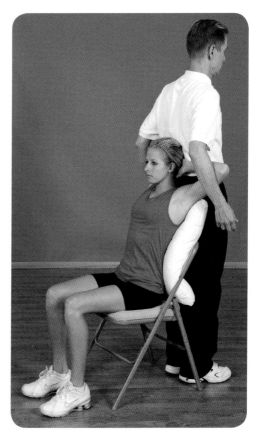

Questions for Self-Reflection

Now that you have had the opportunity to practise some of the stretches shown in chapters 5, 6 and 7, it might be worth reflecting on the following questions:

- In which of the three treatment positions did you prefer to apply your passive stretches: prone, supine or seated?

- Were there any stretches you found particularly easy? Were there any stretches you found particularly challenging? If so, what was challenging about them? Could you modify your position or handhold, the position of the client or the stretch itself to make the stretch effective yet easier to apply?

- How easy was it for your client to relax in order to let you apply passive stretches?

- Can you think of any clients for whom the stretches shown in chapters 5, 6 and 7 might be particularly helpful?

- If you had to advise another therapist in applying passive stretches, what three things do you think are most important to pass along?

Chapter 1

1. Therapeutic stretching is any stretching that is performed with the intention of deliberately facilitating an improvement in a person's physical or psychological well-being.

2. Other treatment interventions include the following:

   Use of ice (cryotherapy)

   Immobilization

   Cognitive behavioural therapy (CBT)

   Manual lymphatic drainage

   Balance training

   Rest

   Exercise

   Massage

3. A sprain is damage to a ligament; a strain is damage to a muscle or its tendon. Both are graded according to their severity—grade I being mild with a few fibres torn, grade III severe (complete rupture), and grade II with more tissue damage than grade I but less than grade III. Both involve pain and swelling, with pain subsiding before tissues are fully healed. Strains tend to heal more quickly than sprains because muscles are more highly vascularized.

4. People stretch

   - to help maintain normal muscle functioning;
   - to help alleviate pain due to muscle tension;
   - to overcome cramping in muscles;
   - to maintain or improve range of motion in a joint;
   - to facilitate muscle healing;
   - to help correct postural imbalances;
   - to help minimize the development of scar tissue; and
   - to influence psychological factors, such as to aid relaxation, maintain or improve motivation or stimulate a sense of well-being.

5. There is no right or wrong answer to this question. All of the points listed within the general safety guidelines are important.

Chapter 2

1. SMART stands for specific, measurable, achievable, realistic and timely.
2. The four types of stretching mentioned are active stretching, passive stretching, muscle energy technique and soft tissue release.
3. When working with elderly patients, it might be better to provide stretches in a seated or lying position because older adults often have problems with balance and decreased strength, so stretches performed in the standing position may be difficult or increase the risk of falls.
4. A goniometer is a device that is used to measure range of motion in joints.
5. Reassessment of clients after stretching is necessary to determine whether the stretching plan has been effective at meeting the goals that were set out.

Chapter 3

1. Active stretches are those that a person performs for himself, without the assistance of a therapist or trainer.
2. Passive stretches are those that require the assistance of another person. This second party—usually a fitness professional, physical therapist or sports massage therapist—is responsible for working in conjunction with a client, positioning the client's body in such a way as to facilitate a stretch.
3. When working with a client for the first time, it is important to provide only one or two easy stretches for the client to perform actively because many people do not heed the advice given them by therapists, and the easier a stretching programme appears to the client, the more likely the client will adhere to it.
4. Both active and passive stretches should be held for a minimum length of 30 seconds.
5. When applying a passive stretch to the limb of a client, you take the limb to the point of mild resistance and hold it there. This is the point at which the client reports a stretch sensation and where there is no pain.

Chapter 4

1. Instruct your client to use up to but not exceed 25 percent of his force when actively contracting a muscle before an MET stretch.
2. The passive stretches described throughout part III can all be used as starting positions for an MET stretch.
3. When applying STR, the muscle being stretched is first shortened and then compressed at various positions along its length as the therapist creates a false origin before lengthening, whereas with MET the muscle to be stretched is usually lengthened before stretching and is not compressed at any point.
4. To lock tissues when using STR, you could use your thumbs, fists, forearms or elbows.

5. Useful books for more information include the following:

   Muscle Energy Techniques by L. Chaitow, Churchill Livingstone (2001)

   Facilitated Stretching by E. McAtee and J. Charland, Human Kinetics (1999)

   Soft Tissue Release by J. Johnson, Human Kinetics (2009)

Chapter 5

1. Active stretches are the most safe for treating sub-acute injuries.

2. It is good to do calf stretches when treating clients with plantar fasciitis because the fascia of the calf connects to the fascia of the foot via the calcaneus, and stretching the calf may help alleviate tension in the plantar fascia.

3. Active stretches are particularly good to recommend to clients suffering calf or hamstring cramps because active contraction of the opposing muscle groups (i.e., the tibialis anterior and quadriceps, respectively) inhibits contraction of the calf and hamstrings.

4. When performing passive adductor stretches in the supine position, it is necessary to prevent the client's pelvis from tilting by placing your hand over the anterior superior iliac spine.

5. To prevent the pelvis from tilting when performing passive stretches to the quadriceps in the prone position, stabilize it by resting on the sacrum.

Chapter 6

1. Swinging the arm in a pendulum-like movement is useful for tractioning the tissues of the shoulder and increasing synovial fluid in the joint, which is helpful for clients with adhesive capsulitis (frozen shoulder).

2. The rationale for incorporating lateral strengthening exercises into a stretching programme for a client with tight internal rotator muscles is that these exercises help inhibit the internal rotators and thus facilitate stretching.

3. With medial and lateral epicondylitis, it is important to keep the elbow extended when performing stretches because both the flexor and the extensor muscles cross the elbow joint, and so keeping the joint extended increases the stretch on these muscles (whereas flexing the elbow reduces the stretch).

4. It is important to also stretch the fingers when helping someone recover from a wrist injury because the tendons of the fingers cross the wrist joint and thus affect its mobility.

5. The four movements of the wrist that need to be regained after a sprain are flexion, extension, radial deviation and ulnar deviation.

Chapter 7

1. When receiving passive neck rotations using a towel, it is better if a client can feel the treatment couch beneath his head because this enables him to relax better.

2. To encourage correct head and neck retraction, a client could be instructed to imagine that she has her chin on a shelf and is drawing it backwards and forwards on this shelf (rather than looking up to the ceiling, which produces neck extension, not retraction).

3. Retracting the scapulae is a simple exercise a client could perform daily to help relax the pectoral muscles.

4. When treating a client for low back strain, the movements of hip hitching should be used before a client is able to bear weight because they may be performed in the supine position.

5. It might be better for a client to perform active rotation of the trunk in a seated position rather than a standing position because in a standing position, clients have a tendency to rotate from the feet, ankles and hips rather than the waist and therefore do not get a proper low back stretch.

Photo Index

LOWER LIMB

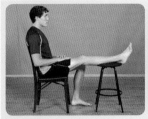

Foot and ankle.
p. 54

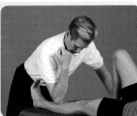

Knee and leg.
p. 63

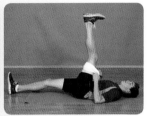

Hip and thigh.
p. 69

UPPER LIMB

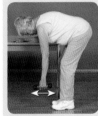

Shoulder.
p. 89

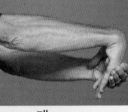

Elbow.
p. 102

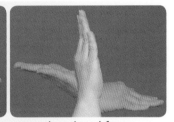

Wrist, hand and fingers.
p. 106

TRUNK

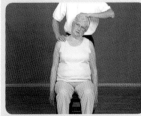

Head and neck.
p. 114

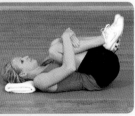

Trunk.
p. 121

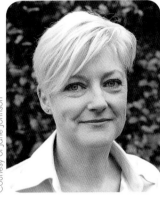

Courtesy of Jane Johnson

Jane Johnson, MSc, is co-director of the London Massage Company (London, England) and is a chartered physio-therapist and sport massage therapist. An experienced body work instructor, Johnson has been a regular provider of continuing professional development workshops for the Federation of Holistic Therapists (FHT) for over 10 years. This experience has brought her into contact with thousands of therapists of all disciplines and helped inform her own practice.

Johnson is also a regular presenter at the annual Complementary and Massage Expo (CAM) held in the United Kingdom. She is a full member of the Chartered Society of Physiotherapists and is registered with the Health Professions Council. She is also a member of the Institute of Anatomical Sciences.

In her spare time, Johnson enjoys taking her dog for long walks, practicing wing chun kung fu, and visiting museums. She resides in London.

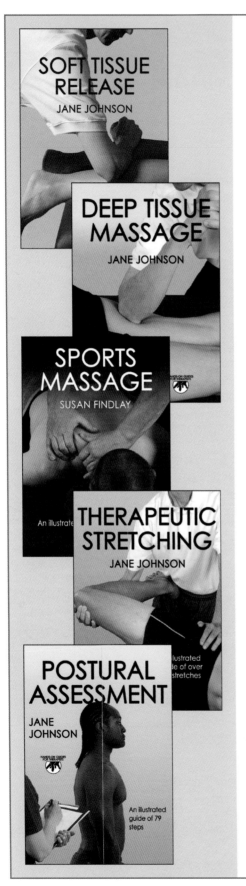
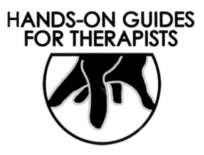